Preface

Hypothermia was first applied to the human in 1940 by *Smith* and *Fay* in an attempt to affect the growth of malignant tumours, and found its most important application firstly in open cardiac surgery and latterly in neurosurgery. The first results regarding the use of hypothermia in neurosurgery were reported at the First International Congress of Neurological Sciences held in Brussels in 1957. The same subject was again considered at the annual meeting of the Société de Neurochirurgie de Langue Française held in Montpellier in 1962.

When I was charged with the task of organizing the Symposium at the Second European Congress of Neurosurgery, I thought it advisable to put forward again the problem of the use of hypothermia in neurosurgery. Though this procedure had rapidly become popular and a mass of publications from the most important neurosurgical centres of the world had appeared, many problems remained unsolved, and in particular those related to the choice of cases to be treated, the usefulness of the procedure and its possible dangers.

In accepting the task of organizing a Symposium on Hypothermia in Neurosurgery, I decided to ask for the collaboration of all those authors who had been the main contributors to the study of the problem, both with clinical and experimental research. I decided to entrust Dr. *Rosomoff* of Pittsburg, U.S.A., with the problem of the physiopathology of the nervous system during the hypothermic state; Professor *Kristiansen* of Oslo, Norway, with the problem of selective hypothermia; Drs. *Michenfelder* and *Uihlein* of the Mayo Clinic, Rochester, U.S.A., with the problem of deep hypothermia and Drs. *Lazorthes* and *Campan* of Toulouse, France, with the problem of hypothermia in post-operative care and cranial trauma.

I reserved for myself and the staff of the neurosurgical Clinic of Milano the task of dealing with the technical details, anaesthetic management, indications and contra-indications and results of moderate hypothermia in neurosurgery.

I hope that the data set out in these reports and the discussions included in the papers will give a clear account of the present position of hypothermia in neurosurgery.

I was aware of the fact that my request to the contributors to this Symposium involved considerable effort on their part, for which I wish to thank them and I was greatly honoured that so many distinguished workers agreed to contribute papers on this subject.

Milano, July 1964

P. E. Maspes

Contents

ACTA NEUROCHIRURGICA / SUPPLEMENTUM XIII

HYPOTHERMIA IN NEUROSURGERY

SYMPOSIUM ORGANIZED BY P. E. MASPES
AT THE
SECOND EUROPEAN CONGRESS OF NEUROSURGERY
ROME, APRIL 18—20, 1963

EDITED BY

P. E. MASPES AND B. HUGHES
MILANO   BIRMINGHAM

WITH 67 FIGURES

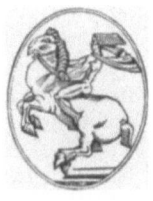

1964

SPRINGER-VERLAG / WIEN · NEW YORK

ISBN-13:978-3-211-80683-8   e-ISBN-13:978-3-7091-5474-8
DOI:10.1007/978-3-7091-5474-8

Titel Nr. **9120**

I. Pathophysiology of Hypothermia

Reparto Neurochirurgico — Ospedale Civico e Benfratelli — Palermo (Italy)

General Physiology of Hypothermia

By

M. Rossanda

With 3 Figures

The present paper neither represents a personal contribution to physiology of hypothermia, nor is it a complete review of the respiratory, circulatory and metabolic changes observed in hypothermia. An effort has been made to give a simple picture of the main physiologic alterations.

It is important to distinguish between alterations produced by the lowered temperature and those dependent upon the body's reaction to cooling. When the response to cooling is completely inhibited, as in deep anaesthesia, lowering of the internal temperature is followed by a simultaneous and progressive depression of the respiratory and circulatory functions. In this case, however, anaesthesia itself may contribute to depression; in fact the respiratory and circulatory failure can be precipitated when deep anaesthesia is used in order to facilitate the induction of hypothermia.

On the other hand, when the cooling procedure is performed under too light anaesthesia, intense vasoconstriction, shivering and epinephrine discharges are likely to occur. A picture of strong respiratory, circulatory and metabolic stimulation becomes evident, which is totally opposite to that just described. The danger is now as great as in the case of excessive depression.

In the Figs. 1 and 2, an attempt has been made to emphasize graphically the concept just exposed. The curves of the diagrams have no mathematical background, nor are they originated from a personal experience. They express average pictures resulting from the literature.

The Fig. 1 shows the general course of respiratory changes during cooling. When the temperature regulating mechanisms are fully inhibited, the entire body oxygen consumption falls as the body temperature decreases. In the presence of shivering, instead, the oxygen uptake may be much greater than normal even when the internal temperature is lowered (*Dill* and *Forbes*, 1941; *Bigelow* et al., 1950). At 30° C this metabolic response to cooling is still present; it disappears only around 20° C (*Kuznetsova*, 1960).

In other words, during mild hypothermia, the oxygen consumption is reduced to about 50% when the level of anaesthesia has been carefully controlled; however, a sudden rise in metabolic

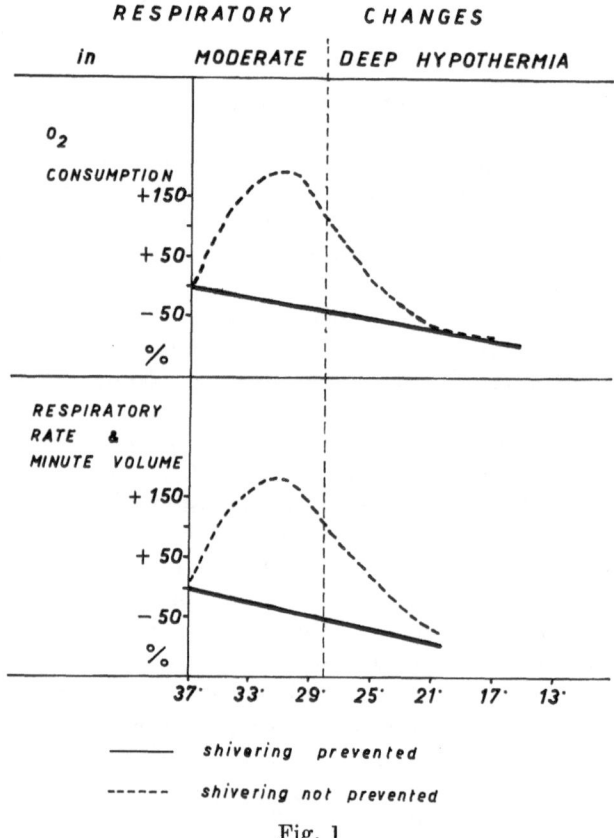

Fig. 1

rate may still follow the inadvertent reduction of the depth of anaesthesia. In deep hypothermia, on the contrary, oxygen consumption is reduced to about 10—15% and no further anaesthetic is required in order to avoid shivering and rise of the metabolic rate (*Giaja*, 1953; *Fisher* et al., 1955).

When the hypothermic state is maintained for many hours, the oxygen consumption does not vary. During the rewarming phase, the oxygen uptake may be equal (*Bigelow* et al., 1950) or higher (*Kuznetsova*, 1960) to that observed at the same temperature before the induction of hypothermia. A larger consumption in the rewarming phase may represent the payment of a debt of oxygen. In fact, hypothermia per se does not expose the body to anoxia*, but when shivering or vasoconstriction are left to manifest themselves during the hypothermic state, a large amount

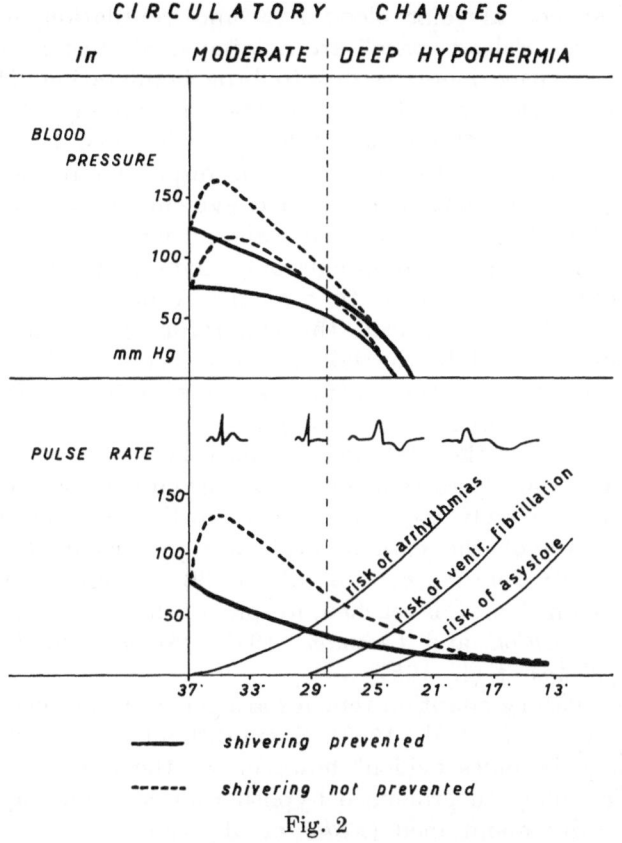

Fig. 2

* It seems to me that most Authors are in agreement that the shift of the dissociation curve of haemoglobin in hypothermia is of no practical value or significance. In fact, this shift means that oxygen bound to Hb can be taken up by the tissues only after a low level of pO_2 has been reached. However, during the cooling, an increase of the plasma oxygen solubility and a drop of the oxygen requirement takes place simultaneously. In deep hypothermia, when the shift effect becomes important, the entire requirement of oxygen could be supplied by the amount dissolved in the plasma (*Dill* and *Forbes*, 1941; *Penrod*, 1951; *Rosenhain* and *Penrod*, 1951).

of tissues (muscle, skin) can contract an oxygen debt, that will
be offset in the rewarming phase.

The respiratory minute volume and rate follow generally the
line of the oxygen consumption (*Blair* and *Fellows*, 1960). However, around 20° C the medullary centres are directly inhibited
and the breathing stops. This is a reversible phenomenon (*Golovin*,
1960; *Klykov*, 1960).

In mild hypothermia the gas exchange in the lung and the
relation between alveolar blood flow and ventilation, expressed
by the "alveolar dead space" are not impaired. Instead the anatomical dead space increases due to bronchodilatation. The com-
pliance does not vary; the intrapulmonary mixing of gases is
moderately slowed (*Otis* et al., 1957; *Severinghaus*, 1959).

At 30° C the respiratory centre is still responsive to the changes
in blood pCO_2; in fact, there is good evidence that hypercapnia
in the cooling originates from anaesthetic depression.

In Graph 2 the main circulatory changes are shown. The
general course is similar to that of the respiratory alterations.
It is, however, not identical; the respiratory depression is progressive and parallel to the fall of the oxygen requirment. The
circulatory changes, on the contrary, are less continuous (*Hamilton*
et al., 1937; *Juvenelle* et al., 1952).

Down to 28° C the systolic and diastolic blood pressure and
the cardiac output decrease moderately. The circulation is generally
adequate to the body requirment. The cardiac rhythm is slowed
and all phases of the cardiac cycle are prolonged (*Forlivesi* e
Naldini, 1959; *Emslie-Smith* et al., 1959). Severe arrhythmias
occur rarely until 28° C is reached, in spite of the increase in cardiac
irritability* (*Elliott* and *Crismon*, 1947; *Covino* and *Hegnauer*,
1956; *Angelakos* et al., 1957).

The circulatory adaption reflexes are generally preserved down
to 30—28° C (*Blair* et al., 1959). Some difficulty in compensating
haemorrhage becomes evident however, as the temperature falls
(*Simkhovic*, 1960). In prolonged hypothermia a circulatory steady
state is hardly maintained (*Fedor* et al., 1958).

Below 28° C all circulatory functions are severely threatened.
The blood pressure drops, and cardiac arrhythmias occur fre-

---

* In neurosurgical hypothermia, where cardiac manipulation does not
take place, two possible sources of cardiac arrhythmias are taken in account:
a) stimulation of nervous structures near the diencephalon (*Purpura* et al.,
1958; *Pool* and *Kessler*, 1958) and b) temperature gradients between cardiac
cavities, which can be large enough during the rapid blood stream cooling
(*Sweet* et al., 1959).

quently, there is great risk of ventricular fibrillation (*Schlosser* and *Grote*, 1962; *Stephen* et al., 1961; *Starkov*, 1960).

In fact, the limit between mild and deep hypothermia (28° C) should not be passed without extracorporeal circulation.

When the internal temperature falls to 20° C, the risk of cardiac asystole becomes very great; vasomotor activity is no longer detectable. Cardiac asystole and vasomotor inhibition are both spontaneously reversible in the rewarming (*Golovin*, 1960; *Klykov*, 1960). In many instances, however, the heart does not start rhythmically but fibrillates (*Stephan* et al., 1961).

With reference to the mechanism of hypothermic ventricular fibrillation, no agreement has been reached to date (*Montgomery* et al., 1954; *Swan* et al., 1955; *Niazi* and *Lewis*, 1956; *Shumacker* et al., 1956; *Boeré*, 1957; *Margolis*, 1958; *Anlyan* et al., 1958; *Kolb* et al., 1959; *Pokrovskij* and *Bensman*, 1960; *Osborne* et al., 1961; *Covino* and *D'Amato*, 1962; *Ebert* et al., 1962). Several preventing drugs have been tested. None have proved capable of reducing constantly the incidence of ventricular fibrillation in hypothermia, with the possible exception of high doses of quinidine (*Angelakos* and *Hegnauer*, 1959).

Methods of preventing ventricular fibrillation in cooling and rewarming are being tested, in order to permit neurosurgery under deep hypothermia without opening the thorax (*Woodhall* et al., 1960; *Descotes* et al., 1961).

The Fig. 3 shows the effect of cooling on the acid-base balance of the blood plasma (*Brewin* et al., 1955, 1956; *Bradley* et al., 1956; *Severinghaus* et al., 1956; *Axelrod* and *Bass*, 1956).

The cold alters the dissociation of the protein buffers and renders available an amount of base for combining with carbonic acid. When a sample of blood is cooled in a syringe, its bicarbonate content increases at the expense of the dissolved carbon dioxide; because of the greater solubility of the gas, a great reduction in the partial pressure of carbon dioxide will take place; the pH rises. If the blood is cooled in the presence of a steady pCO_2 (in a tonometer), dissolved carbon dioxide and bicarbonate both increase and the pH does not vary.

Blood in whole body, in presence of a steady alveolar pCO_2, is like the latter example. The alveolar pCO_2 is still, under hypothermia, a determinant feature of the blood pH. When the patient is hyperventilated, the blood pH raises during the cooling and the bicarbonate content of the plasma shows a moderate increase.

However, several reports have appeared about the "acidosis of hypothermia". This is metabolic in origin, as shown by the

reduction in the bicarbonate content of the plasma. A mild metabolic acidosis is often detectable during the hypothermic state;
more severe metabolic acidosis has been described as occurring in
the rewarming phase.

Possible sources of hypothermic acidosis are: impaired glucose

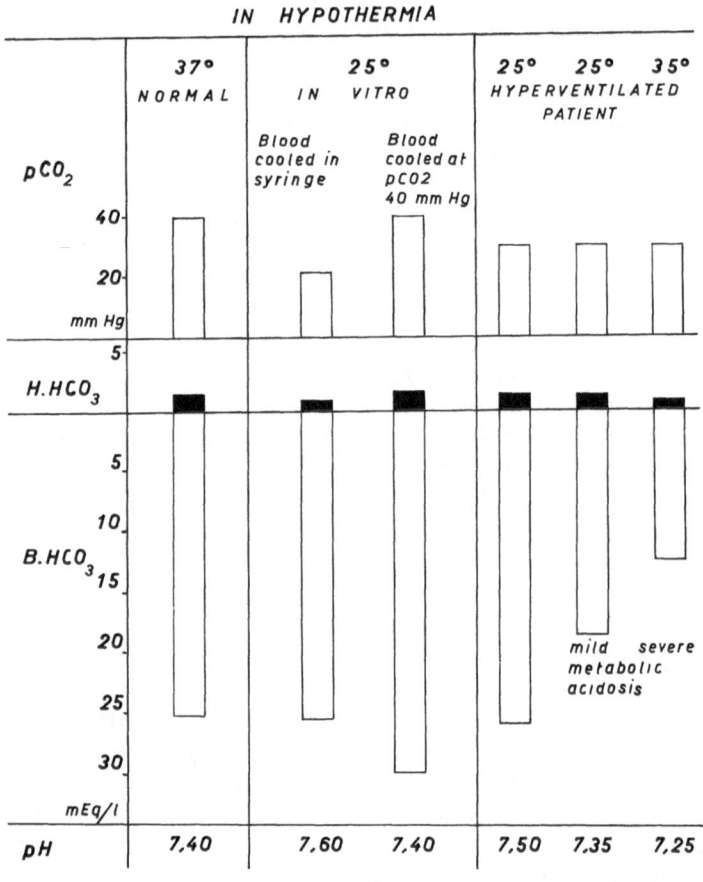

Fig. 3

metabolism (*Wynn*, 1954); citrated blood transfusion (*Henneman*
et al., 1958; *Hara* et al., 1961); anoxia dependent upon arrest of
the circulation (*Neil*, 1957) or low blood flow in extracorporeal
circulation (*Bernhard* et al., 1961); high lactic-acidaemia from
shivering (*Deterling* et al., 1955; *Waddell* et al., 1957), from temperature imbalance between liver and muscle (*Ballinger* et al., 1961),

from excessive hyperventilation (*Bozza Marrubini*, 1963); a temporary reduction of the acid-base regulating activity of the kidney with retention of acid metabolites (*Morales* et al., 1957; *Segar*, 1958; *Terblanche* et al., 1961).

In the blood of hypothermic animals the buffer capacity is decreased because protein buffers are partially substituted by the less efficient bicarbonate buffer. The occurrence of metabolic acidosis renders it more difficult to compensate hypercapnia.

In conclusion, it can be said that, as the temperature falls, the tolerance of the body to the lack of oxygen increases, but at the same time the tolerance to deviations from the normal circulatory and metabolic balance is reduced.

Summary

The main respiratory, circulatory and acid-base alterations occurring in hypothermia are described. Shivering is a very important factor in altering the physiologic pattern of mild hypothermia. Circulatory and metabolic changes are responsible for reduced safety of hypothermic anaesthesia.

Zusammenfassung

Beschreibung der wesentlichen Veränderungen von Atmung, Kreislauf und des Säure-Basen-Verhältnisses während Hypothermie. Frierreaktionen sind ein wesentlicher Faktor für Änderungen der physiologischen Verhältnisse unter gemäßigter Hypothermie. Kreislauf- und Stoffwechselveränderungen sind verantwortlich für eine verminderte Sicherheit der Unterkühlungsnarkose.

Résumé

Les principales altérations respiratoires, circulatoires, et acido basique, survenant dans l'hypothermie sont décrites. Le tremblement est un très important facteur d'altération du comportement physiologique de l'hypothermie modérée. Des modifications circulatoires et métaboliques sont responsables d'une diminution de la sécurité de l'anesthésie hypothermique.

Riassunto

Nel descrivere le principali alterazioni dell'equilibrio respiratorio, circolatorio ed acido-base osservate in ipotermia, l'A. mette in rilievo come il brivido influenzi notevolmente l'andamento delle alterazioni fisiologiche durante l'ipotermia moderata e conclude che nell'anestesia ipotermica vi è una riduzione del margine di sicurezza, dovuta alle alterazioni circolatorie e metaboliche.

Resumen

Se describe las alteraciones principales de la respiración, circulación y del equilibrio acídobásico bajo la hipotermia. El temblór es un factor muy importante respeto a la alteración del curso fisiologico en la hipotermia moderada. Las modificaciones circulatorias y metabolicas son responsables para una disminuición de la seguridad en la anestesia bajo hipotermia.

References

Angelakos, E. T., S. Deutsch, and *L. Williams:* Sensitivity of Hypothermic Myocardium to Calcium. Circulation Res. *5* (1957), 196—201. — *Angelakos, E. T.,* and *A. H. Hegnauer:* Pharmacological Agents for the Control of Spontaneous Ventricular Fibrillation under Progressive Hypothermia. J. Pharmacol. Ther. *127* (1959), 137—145. — *Anlyan, F., E. P. Hastings,* and *E. T. Angelakos:* Comparison of Anesthetics on Incidence of Ventricular Fibrillation in Experimental Hypothermic Ventriculotomy. Anesthesiology *19* (1958), 213—216. — *Axelrod, D. R.,* and *D. E. Bass:* Electrolytes and Acid-Base Balance in Hypothermia. Am. J. Physiol. *186* (1956), 31—34. — *Ballinger, W. F., H. Vollenweider, J. Y. Templeton,* and *L. Pierucci:* Acidosis of Hypothermia. Ann. Surg. *154* (1961), 517—523. — *Bernhard, W. F., S. E. Carroll, H. F. Schwartz,* and *R. E. Gross:* Metabolic Alterations Associated with Profound Hypothermia and Extracorporeal Circulation in the Dog and Man. J. Thor. Card. Surg. *42* (1961), 793—803. — *Bigelow, W. G., W. K. Lindsay, R. C. Harrison, R. A. Gordon,* and *W. F. Greenwood:* Oxygen Transport and Utilisation in Dogs at Low Body Temperature. Am. J. Physiol. *160* (1950), 125—137. — *Blair, E., R. Zimmer,* and *L. Martin:* Haemodynamic Effects of Total Circulatory Occlusion During Hypothermia. Surg. Gyn. Obst. *108* (1959), 13—18. — *Blair, E.,* and *J. Fellows:* Pulmonary Ventilation in Hypothermia. J. Thor. Card. Surg. *39* (1960), 305—311. — *Boba, A.:* Hypothermia for the Neurosurgical Patient. Springfield, Illinois: Thomas. 1960. — *Boeré, L. A.:* Ventricular Fibrillation in Hypothermia. Anaesthesia *12* (1957), 299—310. — *Bozza Marrubini, M.:* personal communication, 1963. — *Bradley, A. F., M. Stupfel,* and *J. W. Severinghaus:* Effect of Temperature on pCO_2 and pO_2 of Blood in Vitro. J. appl. Physiol. *9* (1956), 201—204. — *Brewin, E. G., R. P. Gould, F. S. Nashat,* and *E. Neil:* Investigation of Problems of Acid-Base Equilibrium in Hypothermia. Guy's Hosp. Rep. *104* (1955), 177—214. — *Brewin, E. G., F. S. Nashat,* and *E. Neil:* Acid-Base Equilibrium in Hypothermia. Brit. J. Anaesth. *28* (1956), 2—12. — *Cooper, K.,* and *D. Ross:* Hypothermia in Surgical Practice. London: Cassell. 1960. — *Covino, B. G.,* and *A. H. Hegnauer:* Hypothermic Ventricular Fibrillation and its Control. Surgery *40* (1956), 475—480. — *Covino, B. G.,* and *H. E. D'Amato:* Mechanism of Ventricular Fibrillation in Hypothermia. Circulation Res. *10* (1962), 148—155. — *Descotes, J., J. de Rougemont, P. George,* and *C. Quincy:* L'hypothermie profonde, 10° degrées C., sans thoracotomie — méthode de Gollan-Sealy. Ann. Chir. *15* (1961), 1201—1208. — *Deterling, R. A., Jr., E. Nelson, S. Bhonslay,* and *W. Howland:* Study of Basic Physiologic Changes Associated with Hypothermia. Arch. Surg. *70* (1955), 87—94. — *Dill, D. B.,* and *W. H. Forbes:* Respiratory and Metabolic Effects of Hypothermia. Am. J. Physiol. *132* (1941), 685—697. — *Ebert, P. A., L. J. Greenfield, W. G. Austen,* and *A. G. Morrow:* The Relationship of Blood pH During Profound Hypothermia to Subsequent Myocardial Function. Surg. Gyn. Obst. *114* (1962), 357—362. — *Elliott, H. W.,* and *J. M. Crismon:* Increased Sensitivity of Hypothermic Rats to Injected Potassium and the Influence of Calcium, Digitalis and Glucose on Survival. Am. J. Physiol. *151* (1947), 366—372. — *Emslie-Smith, D., G. E. Sladden,* and *G. R. Stirling:* The Significance of Changes in Electrocardiogram in Hypothermia. Brit. Heart J. *21* (1959), 343—351. — *Fedor, E. J., B. Fisher,* and *S. H. Lee:* Rewarming Following Hypothermia of Two to Twelve Hours. I. Cardiovascular Effects. Ann. Surg. *147* (1958), 515—530. — *Fisher, B., C. Russ, E. Fedor, R. Wilde, P. Engstrom, J. Happel,* and *P. Prendergast:* Experimental Evaluation of Prolonged Hypothermia. Arch. Surg. *71* (1955), 431—448. — *Forlivesi, L.*, and *G. Naldini:* Osservazioni elettrocardiografiche durante ipotermia sperimentale. Min. Anestesiologica *25* (1959), 265—268. — *Giaja, J.:* Sur la physiologie de l'organisme refroidi. Presse Méd. *61* (1953), 128—129. — *Golovin, A. P.:* Changes in Respiration and Arterial Pressure Produced by the Perfusion of a Cold Fluid through the Cerebral Ventricles. pag. 53, *Starkov:* The Problem of Acute Hypothermia. London: Pergamon Press. 1960. — *Hamilton, J. B., M. Dresbach,* and *R. S. Hamilton:* Cardiac Changes During Progressive Hypothermia. Am. J. Physiol. *118* (1937), 71—76. — *Hara, M., J. E. Doherty,* and *G. D. Williams:* Citric Acid Metabolism in the Hypothermic Dog. Surgery *49* (1961), 734—742. — *Henneman, D. H., J. P. Bunker,* and *W. R. Brewster:* Immediate Metabolic Responses to Hypothermia in Man. J. appl. Physiol. *12* (1958), 164—168. — *Juvenelle, A., J. Lind,* and *C. Wegelius:* Quelques possibilités offertes par l'hypothermie générale profonde provoquée. Presse Méd. *60* (1952), 973—978. — *Klykov, N. N.:* Changes in Respiration and Arterial Pressure Produced by the Direct Effect of Low Temperature in the Bulbar Centres. pag. 62, *Starkov:* The Problem of Acute Hypothermia. London: Pergamon Press. 1960. — *Kolb, E., K. Spohn, J. Heinzel,* und *R. Kratzert:* Anaesthesie bei Hypothermie unter 20° im Tierversuch. Anaesthesist *8* (1959), 5. — *Kuznetsova, Z. P.:* Changes in the Process of Gas Exchange in Rabbits as a Result of Single and Multiple Overcooling. pag. 93, *Starkov:* The Problem of Acute Hypothermia. London: Pergamon Press. 1960. — *Margolis, R. N.:* Physiologic Changes in Hypothermia and the Problem of Hypothermic Ventricular Fibrillation. Bull. Insts. New England Medical Center *4* (1958), 151—158. — *Montgomery, A. V., A. E. Prevedel,* and *M. Swan:* Prostigmine Inhibition of Ventricular Fibrillation in the Hypothermic Dog. Circulation *10* (1954), 721—727. — *Morales, P., W. Carbery, A. Morello,* and *G. Morales:* Alterations in Renal Function During Hypothermia in Man. Ann. Surg. *145* (1957), 488—499. — *Neil, E.:* Sequelae of Circulatory Arrest During Hypothermia, Proc. Royal Soc. Med. *50* (1957), 75—83. — *Niazi, S. A.*, and *F. J. Lewis:* Profound Hypothermia in the Dog. Surg. Gyn. Obst. *102* (1956), 98—106. — *Osborn, J. J., F. Gerbode, J. B. Johnson, J. K. Ross, T. Ogata,* and *W. J. Kerth:* Blood Chemical Changes in Perfusion Hypothermia for Cardiac Surgery. J. Thor. Card. Surg. *42* (1961), 462—474. — *Otis, A. B.*, and *J. Jude:* Effect of Body Temperature on Pulmonary Gas Exchange. Am. J. Physiol. *188* (1957), 355—359. — *Penrod, K. E.:* Cardiac Oxygenation during Severe Hypothermia in Dog. Am. J. Physiol. *164* (1951), 79—85. — *Pokrovskij, V. M.*, and *V. M. Bensman:* The Prevention of Ventricular Fibrillation, pag. 166, *Starkov:* The Problem of Acute Hypothermia. London: Pergamon Press. 1960. — *Pool, J. L.*, and *L. A. Kessler:* Mechanism and Control of Centrally Induced Cardiac Irregularities during Hypothermia. J. Neurosurg. *15* (1958), 52—64. — *Purpura, D. P., J. L. Pool, E. M. Housepian, M. Girado, S. A. Jacobson,* and *R. J. Seymour:* Hypothermic Potentiation of Centrally Induced Cardiac Irregularities. Anesthesiology *19* (1958), 27—37. — *Rosenhain, F. R.*, and *K. E. Penrod:* Blood Gas Studies in the Hypothermic Dog. Am. J. Physiol. *166* (1951), 55—61. — *Schlosser, V.*, and *G. Grote:* Veränderungen der Blutgase, des Säure-Basen-Gleichgewichtes und der Kreislaufgrößen bei tiefer Hypothermie unter 20° C im Tierversuch. Thoraxchirurgie *9* (1962), 476—487. — *Segar, W. E.:* Effect of Hypothermia on Tubular Transport Mechanism. Am. J. Physiol. *195* (1958), 91—96. — *Severinghaus, J. W., M. Stupfel,* and *F. Bradley:* Variations of Serum Carbonic Acid pK' with pH and Temperature. J. Appl. Physiol. *9* (1956), 197—200. — *Severinghaus, J. W.:* Respiration in Hypothermia. Ann. New York Acad. Sc. *80* (1959), 384—394. — *Shumacker, H. B., Jr., A. Riberi, R. D. Boone,* and *H. Kayikuri:* Ventricular Fibrillation in the Hypothermic State. The Role of Extrinsic Cardiac Innervation. Ann. Surg. *143* (1956), 223—229. — *Simkhovic, E. J.:* Haemodynamics under Hypothermia in Animals which have Suffered Loss of Blood, pag. 183, *Starkov:* The Problem of Acute Hypothermia. London: Pergamon Press. 1960. — *Starkov, P. M.:* The Problem of Acute Hypothermia. London: Pergamon Press. 1960. — *Stephen, C. R., S. J. Dent, K. D. Hall,* and *W. W. Smith:* Physiologic Reactions during Profound Hypothermia with Cardioplegia. Anesthesiology *22* (1961), 873—881. — *Swan, H., R. W. Virtue, S. G. Blount, Jr.,* and *L. T. Kircher, Jr.:* Hypothermia in Surgery; Analysis of 100 Clinical Cases. Ann. Surg. *142* (1955), 382—400. — *Sweet, W. H., W. R. Brewster, P. Osgood,* and *J. C. White:* Physiology of the Hypothermic State. Proc. I. Internat. Congress Neurological Sciences, Brussels, 1957, vol. II., 304. London: Pergamon Press. 1959. — *Terblanche, J., L. C. Isaacson, L. Eales,* and *C. N. Barnard:* Renal Function during and Immediately after Profound Hypothermia. Surgery *50* (1961), 869—876. — *Waddell, W. G., H. B. Fairley,* and *W. G. Bigelow:* Improved Management of Clinical Hypothermia Based upon Related Biochemical Studies. Ann. Surg. *156* (1957), 542—559. — *Woodhall, B., W. C. Sealy, K. D. Hall,* and *W. L. Floyd:* Craniotomy under Conditions of Quinidine-Protected Cardioplegia and Profound Hypothermia. Ann. Surg. *152* (1960), 37—44. — *Wynn, V.:* Electrolyte Disturbances Associated with Failure to Metabolize Glucose during Hypothermia. Lancet 2 (1954), 575—578.

Laboratory of Experimental Surgery (Neurological), The University of
Pittsburgh School of Medicine and The Veterans Administration Hospital,
Pittsburgh, Pa. (U.S.A.)

Pathophysiology of the Central Nervous System During Hypothermia*

By

H. L. Rosomoff

With 9 Figures

The hypothermic state may be divided into 4 stages: clinical, surgical, deep or profound, and frozen or supercooled. The clinical stage extends from 35° to 32° C, surgical from 32° to 25° C, deep or profound from 25° to 0° C, and the frozen or supercooled from 0° to −8° C. Each stage has characteristic physiological activities, and each, within prescribed limits, is compatible with survival and restoration of complete integrity upon rewarming. It is clear that the low temperature slows the rate of cellular processes and modifies the action of metabolites and other substances. This is not necessarily harmful, as long as anoxia and chemical imbalance do not develop.

The basic physicochemical considerations in hypothermia relate to the laws governing the dependence of cellular activities and their enzymatic reactions on temperature, ions, metabolites, and drugs [1]. Of particular importance are such interdependent cellular phenomena as excitability, rhythmicity, and contractility. When the temperature is lowered, the rate of activity of each process is reduced in accordance with its temperature coefficient. Therefore, the effectiveness of an interdependent system at a given temperature depends on the relative actual rates of the processes within that system, and their respective temperature coefficients. In terms of temperature coefficient, reactions are classified as having a Q_{10} of 1, 2, or 3, indicating that the rates of reaction involved change in this proportion for a 10° C change in tem-

* This study was supported by Research Grant B-2469 from the National
Institute of Neurological Diseases and Blindness, U. S. P. H. S.

perature. That is, in hypothermia with a reduction of temperature of 10° C, the reaction rate of a given process will decrease by a factor of 1, 2, or 3, depending on its temperature coefficient. In general, metabolic and rhythmical processes have a Q_{10} of 3, contraction a Q_{10} of 2, and most physical processes, such as diffusion, a Q_{10} of 1. Accordingly, when the temperature is lowered, the metabolic and rhythmical processes decrease 2 to 3 times as much as the rate of diffusion of metabolites. Therefore, it is perfectly possible for cardiac rhythm to cease, as it usually does between 10° and 25° C, and cellular activity to continue on to a much lower temperature without ill effect, provided anoxia does not supervene. Thus, the control of induced hypothermia rests on an understanding of the cellular phenomena involved, the susceptibility of the systems to temperature, ions, and drugs, and our ability to regulate artificially the activity of these processes by modifying the cellular environment.

Little is known about the details of metabolic activity during hypothermia, except for studies of oxygen consumption. The measurement of oxygen consumption is a rather gross index of metabolic activity, one which reflects only the mean additive or subtractive state of metabolic systems at the organ, cellular, or molecular level. All workers agree that the oxygen consumption of the brain decreases during hypothermia. However, the precise mathematical function to be ascribed to the decline is a matter of some debate.

Field and his associates, utilizing brain slices, demonstrated a linear relationship between the logarithm of the oxygen consumption and temperature centrigrade between 10° and 37° C [2]. *Rosomoff* and *Holaday*, in the intact dog, found a linear relationship between the actual oxygen consumption and temperature between 25° and 37° C [3]. No further analysis improved the fit of their data. This was accompanied by a corresponding decrease in cerebral blood flow (Fig. 1). *Bering*, in the monkey, demonstrated a similar curve to that of *Field* and associates. The best fit for his data was a linear relationship between the logarithm of the oxygen consumption and the reciprocal of the absolute temperature, an Arrhenius type plot [4].

The mathematical gymnastics notwithstanding, all 3 groups agree that there is no physiological zero for oxygen consumption until all metabolic processes are arrested. This is considered to take place only at temperatures lower than — 80° C. Microorganisms can be brought to this low temperature and maintained indefinitely without deleterious effects; and such is a commonplace laboratory procedure for the microbiologist. However, it has not been possible to cool intact animals with survival to less than $-8°$ C. Reliable data are not available for the temperature range from $0°$ to $10°-20°$ C; so for the present we will have to accept the extrapolation of the plots of Drs. *Field* or *Bering* as being the best approximations. From a practical viewpoint, these data do allow very reasonable estimates of rates of oxygen consumption for clinical usage.

For the past decade, hypothermia has been employed by the cardiovascular and neurological surgeon as an almost routine adjunct to certain forms of surgery. The common denominator of these procedures has been the exclusion of the circulation for

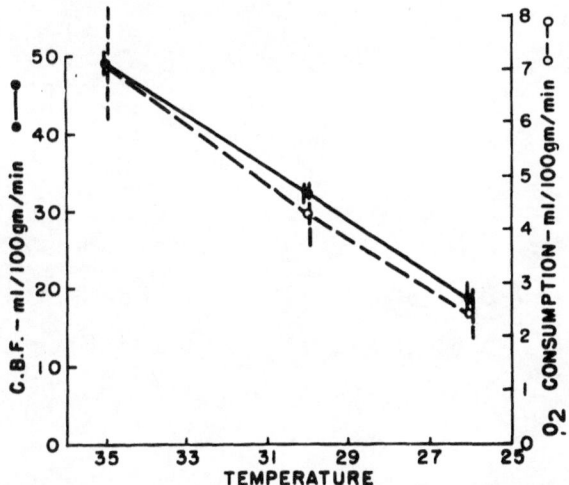

Fig. 1. Cerebral blood and cerebral oxygen during hypothermia.
(From Am. J. Physiol.)

extended periods from the operative field in order to accomplish surgery of the heart or major vessels, which heretofore, was either impossible or most dangerous by conventional normothermic techniques. At $37°$ C, oxygen consumption is unity with a mean tolerable occlusion period of about 5 minutes. At $32°$ C, oxygen consumption is ¾ normal and permits an occlusion of 6—8 minutes. At $28°$ C, consumption is ½ normal with an occlusion period of 10—12 minutes. At $25°$ C, 15—20 minutes are permissible by virtue of a metalobic rate of ⅓. At $10°$ C, 30—45 minutes of cardiac arrest has been tolerated with a metabolic rate of $1/12$. No metabolic data are available for $0°$ and $-8°$ C, but total arrest can be effected for at least 60 minutes.

Along this same avenue of thought, it can be demonstrated
that cerebral infarction can be averted or modified permanently
by hypothermia at the time of, or immediately following, occlusion
of a single artery such as the middle cerebral. The consequence of
interruption of the middle cerebral artery of the dog at normal
body temperature may be seen in Fig. 2. An infarct occurs which
involves the internal capsule, basal ganglia, thalamus, hypo-

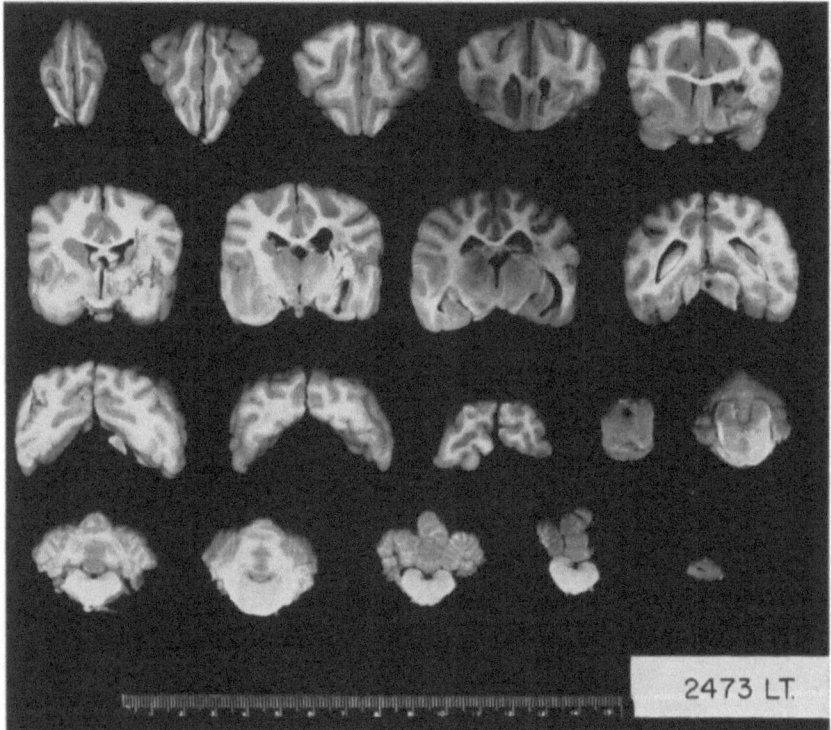

Fig. 2. Coronal sections of a dog brain following transection of the left middle
cerebral artery at normal body temperature. (From the J. Neurosurg.)

thalamus, and portions of the overlying temperoparietofrontal
cortex [5].

By contrast, when the artery is cut during hypothermia, no
infarct occurs or infarction is so slight as to be clinically undetectable.
Such protection can be demonstrated in the animal that is hypothermic at 25° C at the time of transection (Fig. 3).

Protection may also be demonstrated in the animal whose
middle cerebral artery is cut at normal body temperature and then

hypothermia is induced. No signs of infarction are seen, if hypothermia is begun within 15 minutes following transection and if
a temperature of 24° C is reached within a total elapsed time of
90 minutes [6]. Partial protection is afforded if the delay is 15—
30 minutes and the total elapsed time is 90—114 minutes. If either
of these limits is exceeded, no benefit is detectable (Fig. 4).

Unfortunately, the preoccupation with developing techniques

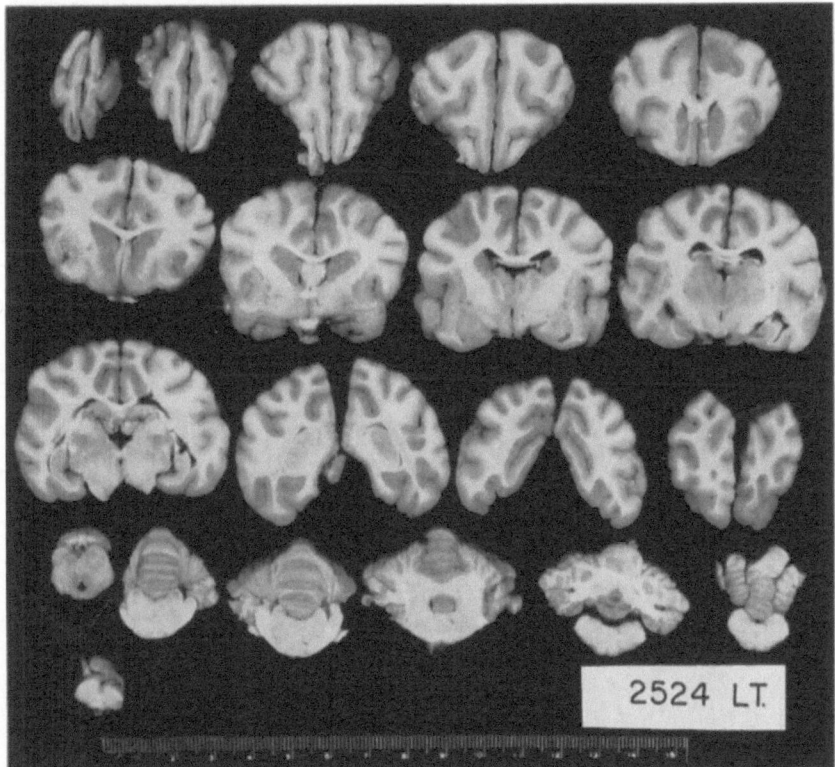

Fig. 3. Coronal sections of a dog brain following transection of the left middle
cerebral artery during hypothermia. (From the J. Neurosurg.)

for successful entry and return from the stage of hypothermia has
overshadowed the collection of physiological data. As such, the
frozen or supercooled stage may be dismissed from discussion with
the statement that small animals like rats and hamsters may be
frozen stiff at —3° C, or supercooled in a limp state to —8° C for
1 hour with survival on rewarming without demonstrable ill effects.
Presumably, the feat is made possible by a drastic depression of

metabolic activity by the cold. Deep or profound hypothermia has also suffered from concern with technique, but, here the major problems have been solved well enough to allow practical daily laboratory and clinical research.

The clinical and surgical stages considered together yield the bulk of the data; but beyond oxygen consumption, there has been no systematic study of the effects of hypothermia on metabolic systems at the cellular or molecular level. Such a project is under way in Pittsburgh with an associate, Dr. *Fred Zugibe*. We have

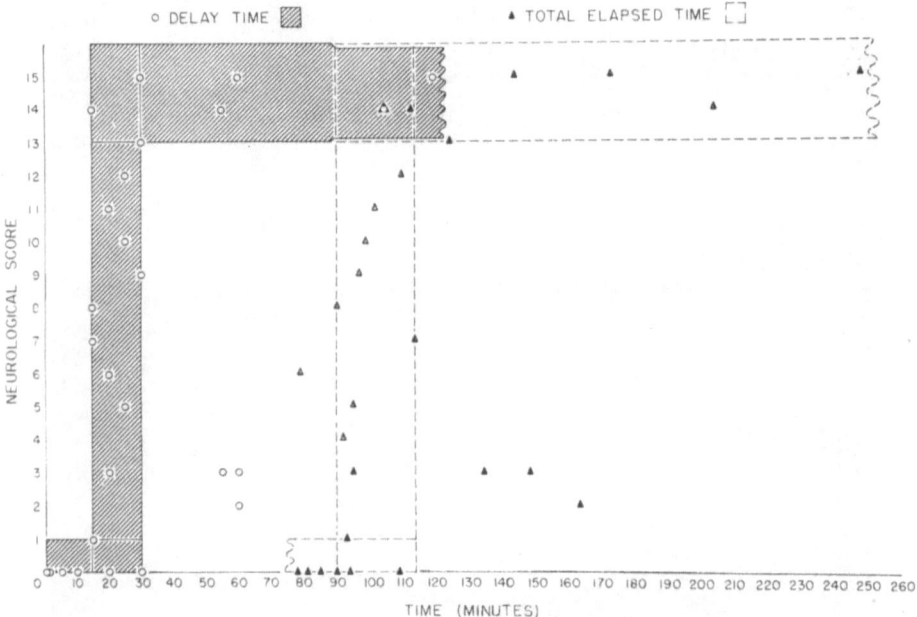

Fig. 4. Effect of hypothermia following interruption of the middle cerebral artery upon the neurological score; the higher the score, the greater the neurological disability. (From the A. M. A. Arch. of Neurol. Psychiat.)

come to a working hypothesis, by no means as yet proved. The experiments were prompted by the following observations. If a brain is injured at normal body temperature, destruction of tissue occurs with the production of a marked inflammatory reaction [7]. As can be seen, the architecture is obliterated and inflammatory congestion is intense (Fig. 5).

By contrast, the same lesion in a hypothermic animal at 25° C, produces pathological changes in the neurons but hardly the devastation seen in the normothermic brain (Fig. 6). Just as im-

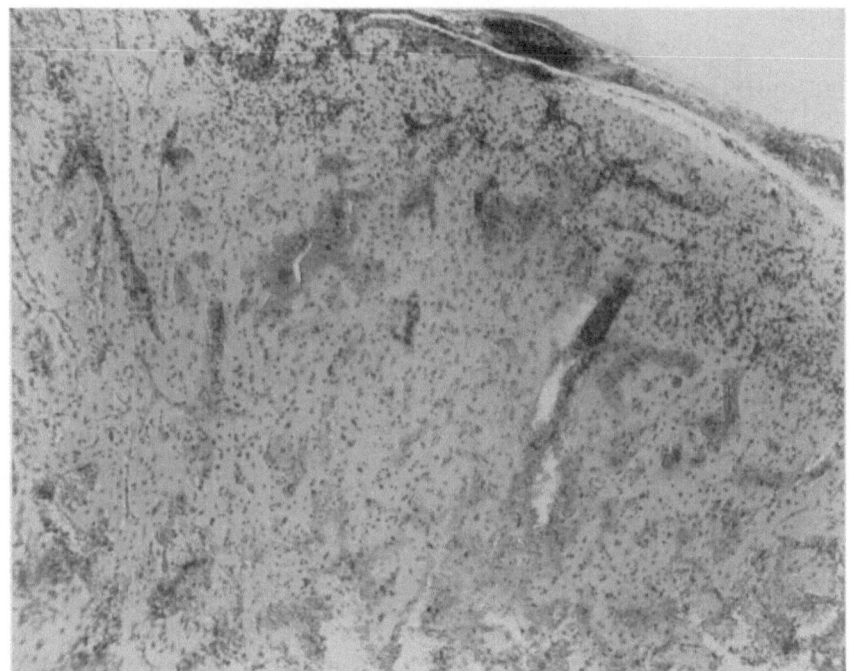

Fig. 5. Microphotograph of a standard brain injury after 12 hours, normal
body temperature. (From the J. Neurosurg.)

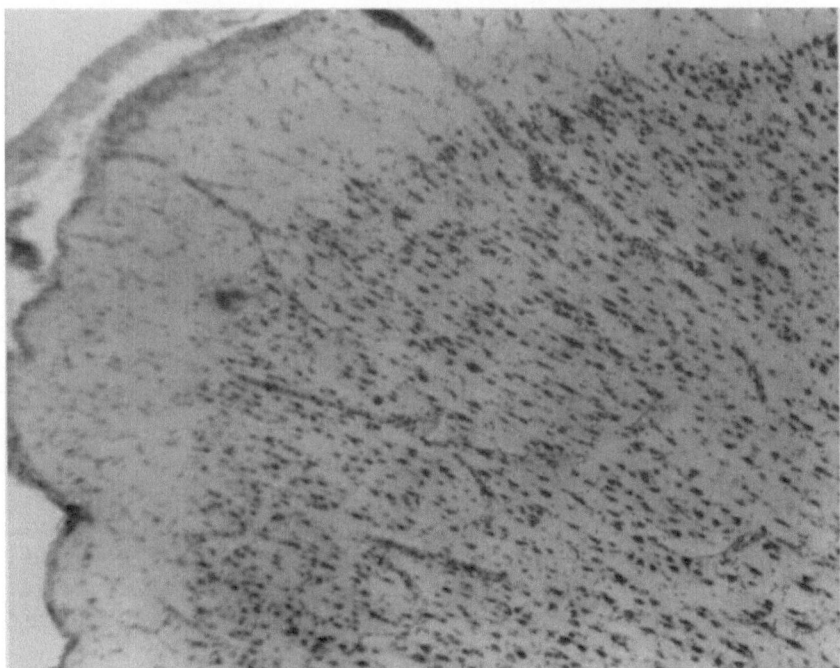

Fig. 6. Microphotograph of a standard brain injury after 12 hours, hypothermia. (From the J. Neurosurg.)

portantly, no cellular inflammatory reaction to injury is found and the development of edema is depressed as long as the animal remains cold. The latter is best seen in Fig. 7. Here equivalent sized lesions were produced in normothermic and hypothermic dogs and the degree of post-traumatic swelling was plotted. The normothermic animals developed progressive, fulminating edema and died. The hypothermic dogs developed a small amount of edema immediately following injury, but thereafter progression was minimal up to 36 hours, the longest period of observation.

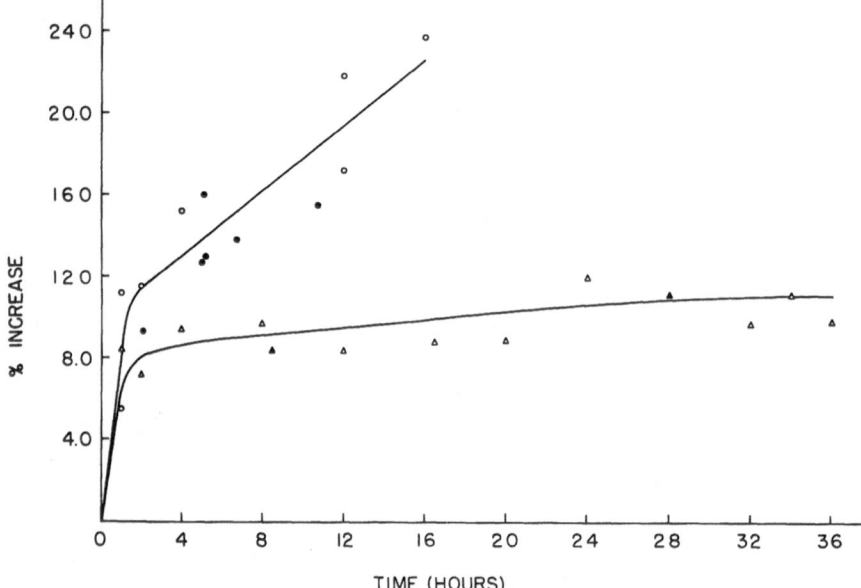

Fig. 7. Graph of the percentage increase of size of the injured hemisphere as compared to the uninjured hemisphere plotted as a function of time. Circles represent normothermic dogs; triangles represent hypothermic dogs, open symbols are animals that were sacrificed; closed symbols are animals that died. (From the J. Neurosurg.)

Reduction of temperature in the uninjured state results in a decrease in brain volume [8]. This, and its compensatory mechanism, is best seen by looking at the distribution of intracranial contents at 25° C. By a new technique, it is possible to determine simultaneously intracranial blood volume, cerebrospinal fluid volume, brain water, and brain solids. It may be seen that at 25° C, the blood volume and brain solids are not altered significantly. However, brain water decreases and this is compensated for by an increase in cerebrospinal fluid volume. It is important to note that the amount of fluid in the head is unchanged; there is no net loss of fluid, only a redistribution occurs (Fig. 8). In finite figures, brain water decreases from a normal of 64.58 percent to 58.92 percent. Cerebrospinal fluid volume increases from 8.92 percent to 13.59 percent, and blood volume and brain solids remain the same. Since there is a reduction of intracellular water and since this is the active force directing the change in cerebrospinal fluid pressure, a decrease in pressure results. This mechanical factor is not the explanation for the decrease in mortality accompanying experimental brain injuries during hypothermia, as will be demonstrated by the following data.

It can be shown that mortality consequent upon brain injury can be prevented if hypothermia is induced within 3 hours of the injury [9]. In this study, a standardized brain injury was utilized that killed 50 percent of a control series of normothermic animals. This size lesion was then produced in an experimental group at normal body temperature followed by the induction of hypothermia at variable times after the injury. If hypothermia was started within 3 hours, all animals survived. If the delay was between 3 and 8 hours, partial protection was afforded. Beyond 8 hours, no benefit was demonstrated. If CSF pressure is measured continuously following such an injury at normal body temperature, there is an immediate sharp rise in the first hour with slowing down thereafter, but reaching a peak in 3 hours (Fig. 9). The pressure remains relatively constant for the ensuing 9 hours. It is interesting that between the third and twelfth hour, there is a sizeable increase in brain volume with little change in pressure. There is no correlation, therefore, between brain size or swelling and pressure under these circumstances. If the same size lesion is produced in another group of animals and hypothermia is induced after 3 hours, there is a characteristic decline in CSF pressure.

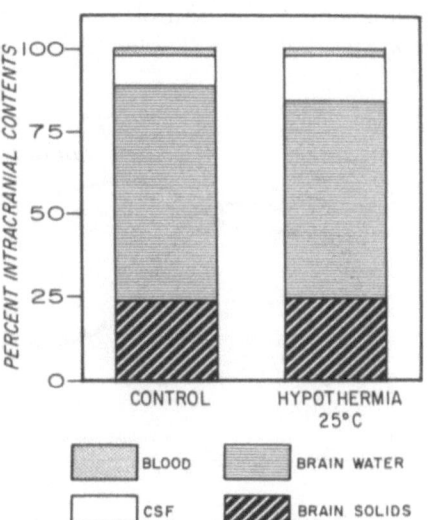

Fig. 8. Distribution of intracranial contents in control dogs and dogs treated with hypothermia

Most interestingly, when hypothermia is discontinued, the pressure reverts to the level seen in untreated animals as if there had never been any change in body temperature. All the hypothermic group survived, 50 percent of the normothermic group died. Therefore, it must be concluded that CSF pressure measurements are of little value either in estimating the rate of survival or the degree of cerebral edema.

At the cellular level, a preliminary series of histochemical studies provide interesting results for speculation. Tissue was obtained from an area of injured brain, adjacent uninjured brain in the same hemisphere, and uninjured brain from the contralateral hemisphere. The samples were analyzed for the content of the enzymes listed in Table 1. The analyses were made in pairs of

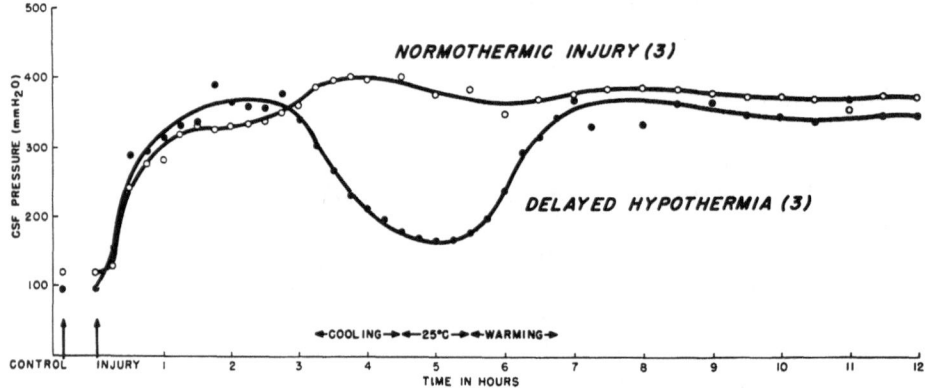

Fig. 9. Cerebrospinal fluid pressure after brain injury at normal body temperature and with delayed hypothermia. (From the Surg., Gyn. Obst.)

normothermic and hypothermic injured dogs at 15, 30, and 60 minute intervals after production of the lesions. There were significant reductions in the amounts of adenosinetriphosphatase, glucose-6-phosphatase, acid phosphatase, and TPNH diaphorase in the injured area of the normothermic animal. This was a local effect in which neither the adjacent or contralateral hemisphere participated. The hypothermic animals showed no alterations in enzyme activity. Each of the affected enzymes is an important member of one or more cellular mechanisms of respiration, as well as being involved in the transport mechanism for water and electrolytes. Adenosinetriphosphatase, for example, is the major source of cellular energy. It is also integral to transport of water and electrolytes through which cellular water balance is maintained. Ordinarily, the cell is hypertonic and requires work to prevent the influx of water. The source of such energy is the high energy phosphate bonds of ATP made available through the activity of ATPase. Therefore, when ATPase is deficient and energy released from ATP is blocked, water is imbibed and the cell swells. Moreover, the enzymes in question are members alone or in combination of the 5 major systems for cellular respiration —

Table 1. *Histoenzymatic Distribution in the Normothermic and Hypothermic Dog Brain One Hour Following Injury*

Enzyme	Normothermic			Hypothermic		
	Injured Area	Area Adjacent to Injury	Opposite Hemisphere	Injured Area	Area Adjacent to Injury	Opposite Hemisphere
Acid Phosphatase	−	+++	+++	+++	+++	++++
Alkaline Phosphatase	++++	++++	++++	++++	++++	++++
Adenosinetriphosphatase	±	+++	+++	+++	+++	+++
Glucose-6-Phosphatase	±	+++	+++	+++	+++	++++
TPNH Diaphorase	+	++	++	++	++	+++
DPNH Diaphorase	++	+++	+++	+++	+++	+++
Succinic Dehydrogenase	++	+++	+++	+++	+++	+++

the glycolytic system, the hexose monophosphate shunt, the Krebs and related cycles for aerobic metabolism, the electron transport system, and the accompanying system for oxidative phosphorylation. Therefore, it appears that hypothermia protects against injury by preventing disruption of cellular respiration and water transport systems. Further research is certainly required along this most promising avenue of investigation.

Summary

Hypothermia is a well-tolerated physiological state whose biophysical properties afford protection against the consequences of cerebral vascular insufficiency and injury.

Zusammenfassung

Hypothermie ist ein gut verträglicher physiologischer Zustand, dessen biophysikalische Eigenschaften einen Schutz bieten gegen die Folgen von zerebrovaskulärer Insuffizienz und von Verletzungen.

Résumé

L'hypothermie est un état physiologique bien toléré et dont les propriétés biophysiques protègent contre les conséquences de l'insuffisance vasculaire cérébrale et les traumatismes.

Riassunto

L'ipotermia è uno stato fisiologico ben tollerato, le cui proprietà biofisiche permettono un'utile protezione contro le conseguenze dell'insufficienza vascolare cerebrale e dei traumi cerebrali.

Resumen

La hipotermia es un estado fisiológico bien tolerado y en el cual las propiedades biofísicas protegen contra las consecuencias que acarrea la insuficiencia vascular cerebral y los traumatismos.

References

1) *Brown, D. E. S.:* Some Considerations of Physiochemical Factors in Hypothermia. The Physiology of Induced Hypothermia. NAS-NRC *451* (1956), 1—7. — 2) *Field, J., F. Fuhrman,* and *A. W. Martin:* Effect of Temperature on the Oxygen Consumption of Brain Tissue. J. Neurophysiol. *7* (1944), 117—126. — 3) *Rosomoff, H. L.,* and *D. A. Holaday:* Cerebral Blood Flow and Cerebral Oxygen Consumption during Hypothermia. Am. J. Physiol. *179* (1954), 85—88. — 4) *Bering, E. A., Jr.:* Effect of Body Temperature Change on Cerebral Oxygen Consumption of the Intact Monkey. Am. J. Physiol. *200* (1961), 417—419. — 5) *Rosomoff, H. L.:* Hypothermia and Cerebral Vascular Lesions: I. Experimental Interruption of the Middle Cerebral Artery during Hypothermia. J. Neurosurg. *13* (1956), 244—255. — 6) *Rosomoff, H. L.:* Hypothermia and Cerebral Vascular Lesions: II. Experimental Middle Cerebral Artery Interruption followed by Induction of Hypothermia. A. M. A. Arch. Neurol. Psychiat. *78* (1957), 454—464. — 7) *Rosomoff, H. L.:* Experimental Brain Injury during Hypothermia. J. Neurosurg. *16* (1959), 177—187. — 8) *Rosomoff, H. L.:* Effect of Hypothermia and Hypertonic Urea on Distribution of Intracranial Contents. J. Neurosurg. *18* (1961), 753—759. — 9) *Rosomoff, H. L., K. Shulman, R. Raynor,* and *W. Grainger:* Experimental Brain Injury and Delayed Hypothermia. Surg. Gyn. Obst. *110* (1960), 27—32.

Clinica Neurochirurgica — Università degli Studi — Milano (Italy)
Service d'Eléctroencéphalographie — Hôpital Neurologique — Lyon (France)

Neurological Observations During Hypothermia

By

C. A. Pagni and J. Courjon

The data which demonstrate that an homoiothermal animal or a man can be refrigerated to low body temperatures without danger and with complete recovery of his thermoregulating capacity are very old. *Peter* (1872) and *Reincke* (1875) reported in the 19th century cases of patients whose internal temperature (rectal) had descended from accidental causes to extremely low points, 24° C — 26° C, and who had recovered. *Simpson* (1902) demonstrated that a monkey cooled to 14° C could survive and recover. *Simpson* and *Herring* (1905) showed that it was possible to take cats down to 16° C and that these recovered if warmed. *Britton* (1923) demonstrated that cats with rectal temperatures of 19° C recover spontaneously.

In spite of these data for a long time it was generally accepted that man could not survive long with an internal temperature below 35°C (*Fay*, 1940), and the internal temperature below which there could be no recovery was held to be relatively high (*Talbott*, 1944).

Mares and *Hellich* back in 1889 had produced a fall in temperature of 3.5° C in a case of hysteria, but it was only in November 1938 that *Fay* refrigerated a patient with a mammary carcinoma to 31°—32° C (*Fay*, 1940), thus opening the period of modern applied hypothermia.

After the experience of *Fay* (*Fay*, 1940; *Fay* and *Smith*, 1941) refrigeration to 26°—31° C was used by other authors as a method of therapy for tumors (*Gerster* et al., 1940; *Talbott*, 1941). Successively other authors used hypothermia for treatment of mental diseases (*Spradley* and *Marin Foucher*, 1949; *Talbott* and *Tillotson*, 1941) and of cranio-cerebral trauma (*Fay*, 1945; *Lazorthes* and *Campan*, 1958).

More recently the use of hypothermia as a complement to anaesthesia for surgical therapy of numerous affections, not only of the central nervous system, has been widely diffused. (See references in the other papers of this symposium.)

In spite of the great number of papers on moderate and deep hypothermia, information on the neurologic and psychiatric modifications induced in the human by the progressive lowering of internal temperature are rather scarce and gathered in two groups of papers:

1) A few papers, going back to about twenty years ago, dealing

with groups of patients on which artificial hypothermia was practiced. The data found in this material are generally limited to the effects of temperatures not lower than 27° C. Only in some cases was the temperature as low as 23°—24° C.

2) Some papers, often very old, in which cases of accidental hypothermia are reported. In this group of papers we can find data regarding patients with lower internal temperature than the previous group (down to 18° C).

Some records of the effects of rapidly induced hypothermia in anaesthetized or non anaesthetized men, in German concentration camps during second world war, have also been reported (*Aléxander*, 1945; *Rosenstiel*, 1946).

Simpson had already demonstrated in 1902 that monkeys cooled with ether anaesthesia to a temperature of 25° C remain in a state of narcosis without further addition of anaesthetics: they are in fact narcotized by cold and in a state of what may be termed "artificial hibernation".

The same happens in the human: once the induction of the narcosis is obtained, for instance with barbiturates, and the temperature reaches 31°—32° C, the patient is semi-asleep and may be maintained in this state with less and less sedation. After the patient has been in state of hypothermia from 8 to 24 hours without any additional sedation, it is reasonable to assume that changes then occurring in reflex activity and consciousness may be due to the effects of refrigeration (*Fay* and *Smith*, 1941).

We will report the neurological modifications which can be assumed to be due only to the lowering of the body temperature.

The data coming from the papers on therapeutic hypothermia and on accidental cooling cover the field and generally agree. Possible discrepancies may be explained by different conditions: duration of exposure to cold; stopping of progressive lowering of the temperature; inevitable anoxia caused by shivering in accidental hypothermia; gradual or rapid fall of the temperature.

Some of the data which we will report were also obtained from the study of 73 patients affected by intracranial aneurysms operated upon under moderate hypothermia, 35 of which were alert, after intervention, at a body temperature of 30—31° C.

The observations on deep hypothermia have been obtained from the study of 75 cases of patients affected by cardiovascular diseases and submitted to operation in deep hypothermia (down to 7° C).

Consciousness and Speech

As the temperature falls the patient becomes increasingly more drowsy and slower in his responses; the lower the temperature the slower is the cerebration of the patient (*Fay* and *Smith*, 1941; *Talbott*, 1944).

Until a rectal temperature of 34° C is reached, the patient may be perfectly alert, cooperative and well oriented, but as the temperature decreases below 33° C the patient is slower in his responses and tends to fall asleep. He becomes clearly dysarthric at 34°—32° C.

However it must be emphasized that at 31°—30° C the patient is generally only sleepy; although sometimes stuporose he is not comatose. He may be awaked from this state by a very light stimulus (a call by voice, a very light touch) and he can speak and answer questions. This is true also for patients just awakened from anaesthesia.

As the temperature falls further, speech becomes dysarthric and tremulous. At 29°—28° C the patient is still able to answer correctly simple questions, but with a very long delay (*Fay* and *Smith*, 1941; *Laufman*, 1951). The speech at this level is clearly dysarthric and often perseveration ensues.

Only *Rees* (1958) reported a patient who, with a rectal temperature of 28° C had no reduction of consciousness, and *Starkow* (1960) reported that a "wounded man . . . . retained consciousness with body temperature of 26°—29° C".

At an even lower temperature, 27° C, it is impossible to obtain vocal responses; the patient grunts when questioned.

Below 26° C the patient is comatose and does not react to any stimulus however strong. (*Peter*, 1872; *Reincke* 1875; *Reinhard*, 1884; *Laufmann*, 1951; *Emslie-Smith*, 1958; *Capron*, 1958; *de Grailly* et al., 1959; *Justin-Besançon* et al., 1960; *Pestel* et al., 1961.) Only *Reincke* (1875) reported the case of a patient who at 27° C still said some words and *Fay* and *Smith* (1941) refered to another one whose conversation still persisted at 23.5° C.

No patient can recall anything that happened during the period of refrigeration below 32° C, although memory and consciousness are partially preserved during cooling between 32° C and 28° C (*Fay* and *Smith*, 1941; *Talbott*, 1941; *Talbott*, 1944; *Gerster* et al., 1940).

Motility

Voluntary movements become progressively slower as the temperature falls.

In our experience some patients at 31° C body temperature

(immediately after the operation, about 6 hours after the induction of anaesthesia with very little Pentothal) performed movements by order (i. e. finger-nose test, etc.) quickly enough and smoothly.

But at lower temperatures, i. e. 30°—28° C, voluntary movements are excessively slow and delayed (*Fay* and *Smith*, 1941; *Rees*, 1958). According to *Fay* and *Smith*, with the body temperature at approximatly 29.5° C the patient requires fifteen to thirty seconds to perform the finger-nose test.

At 30°—28° C the movement is slow, incoordinated, resembling the hypertonic movements of Parkinson's disease (*Fay* and *Smith*, 1941), but no athetotic, dystonic or choreic movements were observed.

At 29°—27° C the patient does not speak and does not move his limbs, but his eyes are open and they follow the examiner or, for instance a moving object (*Meyer* and *Hunter*, 1957; *Laufmann*, 1951).

At temperature of 27° C it is possible to observe reactions to noxious stimuli (*Reincke*, 1875; *Meyer* and *Hunter*, 1957), but at temperatures below 27° C the patient is deeply comatose and does not react any more to any stimulus (*Peter*, 1872; *Reincke*, 1875; *Reinhard*, 1884; *Laufmann*, 1951; *Emslie-Smith*, 1958; *de Grailly* et al., 1959; *Justin-Besançon* et al., 1960).

Deambulation was explored by *Fay* and *Smith* (1941) and *Gerasimenko* (1950): at temperature of 32°—34° C the patient walks unsteadily in a staggering ataxic manner.

Experimental studies have demonstrated that cats and dogs may perform spontaneous skeletal muscle movements at much lower temperature than human beings: *Britton* (1923), *Haterius* and *Hegnauer* (1949) report spontaneous movements in dogs and cats at 20° C and 17° C respectively.

On the other hand the monkey behaves like man according to the results of *Callaghan* et al. (1954), who report reactions to noxious stimuli at 29° C and spontaneous movements at 32° C.

Muscle Tone

If a patient is submitted to refrigeration without premedication very strong shivering develops, which disappears as the temperature falls, giving place to stiffness (*Rosenstiel*, 1946).

With lowering of temperature the muscle tone increases and the muscles assume a waxy stiffness: the upper and lower extremities assume a flexed position and considerable effort is required to extend them. The wrists are flexed; the hands take on a claw-like attitude, with extended metacarpo-phalangeal joints and flexed interphalangeal joints.

The increased muscle tone persists throughout the period of refrigeration.

Fay and *Smith* (1941) describe this attitude and tone in patients with rectal temperatures as low as 26.2° C.

Information concerning muscle tone at temperatures lower than 26.2° C is available only in the papers on accidental hypothermia. At the lowest temperature there is an extreme rigidity with opistothonus. Passive displacement of head and limbs is very difficult (*Peter*, 1872; *Reincke*, 1875; *Laufmann*, 1951; *de Grailly* et al., 1959; *Pestel* et al., 1961). Sometimes the patient has a posture resembling decerebrate rigidity (*de Grailly* et al., 1959) with superimposed hypertonic movements resembling "crises toniques postérieures" (*Justin-Besançon* et al., 1958a, 1960).

Pestel et al. (1961) report that the rigid limbs keep the imposed positions as in catatonia.

Deep Reflexes

Deep reflexes increase with the lowering of the temperature. When the rectal temperature is between 37° C and 32° C deep reflexes are increased. These reflexes become less active when the temperature range is 32° C to 30° C, but at 30° C they are always more active than before the hibernation. Below 30° C the reflexes are more and more reduced and according to *Fay* and *Smith* (1941) the deep reflexes are absent below 26° C. *Reinhard* (1884), *Capron* (1958), *Emslie-Smith* (1958) observed that deep reflexes were still present at 22°—24° C, although very reduced.

According to *Simpson* and *Herring* (1905) and *Britton* (1923) the knee jerk is the last reflex to disappear in cats during cooling, and may be elicited at a rectal temperature of 16° C.

Pestel et al. (1961) believe that the knee jerk is the first reflex to reappear during rewarming in the hypothermic man.

In hypothermia, when the deep reflexes are elicited, the muscles contract very slowly and the time of contraction is prolonged (*Emslie-Smith*, 1958). *Britton* (1923) remarked that the knee jerk reflex, at very low temperatures, takes one to three seconds to subside.

It must be remembered that the period of hyperreflexia corresponds closely to the shivering stage.

Muscle Excitability

Muscle excitability increases in hypothermia: percussion of the muscles causes them to contract slowly.

At low temperatures (29° —24° C) spontaneous or provoked myoclonias (*Fay* and *Smith*, 1941) and facial spasms (*de Grailly* et al., 1959) may be observed.

Pupillary Reflexes

In moderate hypothermia the pupils remain equal and normal in size and react to light stimuli until a temperature of 27° C is reached (*Fay* and *Smith*, 1941). But it must be stressed that pupillary reflexes to light become more and more sluggish as the temperature falls: sometimes at 30°—31° C the pupillary contraction is very slow and so reduced that it may seem to have been lost; at 27° C the pupils require four seconds to reach their maximum contracted state.

Below 27° C the pupillary reflex is generally abolished (*Wayburn*, 1947; *Streit*, 1955; *Emslie-Smith*, 1958; *de Grailly* et al., 1959), but *Emslie-Smith* (1958) observed a very sluggish reflex still at 24° C.

At temperatures lower than 27° C the pupils may be miotic.

The reaction to accomodation is present but very sluggish at 31° C. It was never possible to perform the test for accomodation at lower temperatures.

The Corneal Reflex

The corneal reflex is present down to 27° C, but becomes more sluggish at lower temperatures and disappears altogether at 24°—23° C.

Hoffman Reflex: Clonus

A positive Hoffman's sign may be obtained between 36° C and 30.5° C, i. e. during the phase of increased deep reflexes.

Below 30.5° C the sign, if not present at normal temperature, disappears. The Hoffman sign provoked by lowering of the body temperature is always bilateral.

An ankle clonus may be observed between temperature levels of 36° and 30.5° C, and disappear below 30° C.

Abdominal and Cremasteric Reflexes

The abdominal reflexes remain constant until a temperature of 30.5° C is reached; as the temperature falls they are reduced and finally abolished below 27° C.

The cremasteric reflexes cannot be elicited during hypothermia (*Fay* and *Smith*, 1941).

The Plantar Skin Reflex

According to *Fay* and *Smith* (1941) in no patient does a positive Babinski reaction develop while in hibernation at temperatures as low as 26° C.

In therapeutic moderate hypothermia *Talbott* (1944), *Gerster* et al. (1940), *Meyer* and *Hunter* (1957), did not observe the appearance of a positive Babinski sign in patients who did not display this sign before cooling. However they reported the absence of plantar skin response.

In the review of the literature on accidental hypothermia we have found many cases, in which at very low temperatures (23°—26° C) there was no response or no clear response to plantar stimulation but never a Babinski reflex (*Emslie-Smith*, 1958; *de Grailly* et al., 1959; *Justin-Besançon* et al., 1960; *Pestel* et al., 1961). However *Justin-Besançon* et al. (1960) report a case in which a Babinski reaction developed; the patient died, but the histopathological study of the brain failed to show any lesion.

In short: the plantar skin reflex remains flexor down to 26° C. At lower temperatures the response to plantar stimulation may no longer be present, but, generally, there is never a Babinski reflex.

Neurological Symptoms

Any neurological symptoms that may have been present prior to the induction of hypothermia remain unchanged, under moderate hypothermia, during the whole period of cooling, and subsequently.

During hypothermia, the Babinski reflex, clonus, spasticity, asymmetry of the reflexes etc. can be observed. However, according to our experience, it must be remembered that during hypothermia neurological symptoms are sometimes less easily detectable than at normal body temperature.

We believe that the exact knowledge of the modifications induced by moderate hypothermia on reflex patterns and psychiatric functions is of practical interest to the neurosurgeon.

Immediately after operation patients can be awakened from the anaesthesia at a body temperature of 30°—31° C.

At a rectal temperature as low as 30°—32° C patients are fairly alert: they can answer questions, and perform voluntary movements in response to simple commands. We can affirm that

at a temperature as low as 29°—30° C consciousness is not lost
if the patients are free of anaesthetic. It must be remembered
that at 32°—33° C patients are clearly dysarthric and that their
speech may be indistinct: at this body temperature dysarthria
does not indicate a left temporal lobe lesion. At 34°—31° C the
pupillary reflex to light is very sluggish or quite indistinct: this is
a direct consequence of low body temperature.

Moderate hypothermia *per se* does not provoke, generally,
functional or pathological nervous system damage which can
explain, after rewarming, the appearance of permanent neurologic
disturbances. This point is proved from the studies of *Fay* and
Smith (1941) and from some cases of accidental hypothermia which
after rewarming recovered perfectly.

From our clinical experience it can be said moreover that
moderate hypothermia *per se* does not produce any detectable
lesion of the central nervous system. This belief is based on the pre-
and post-operative study of 73 patients, with intracranial aneurysms
who underwent operation presenting no neurological disturbances
or with stable neurologic signs. In practically every case in whom
postoperative neurologic disturbances were observed, we were able
to indicate some surgical incident, apart from moderate hypothermia, which could explain these changes.

After moderate hypothermia the occurrence of anisocoria,
Babinski, asymmetry of reflexes and of muscle tone, paresis
etc., if not present before the operation, means that cerebral
damage due to the surgical manipulations, took place during the
operation.

On the contrary deep hypothermia may perhaps provoke
per se some neurological disturbances.

In 9 out 75 cases of deep hypothermia (down to 7° C of body
temperature) we observed after the operation choreiform movements (2 cases) and epileptic seizures (7 cases).

Delay et al. (1961), and *Bergouignon* et al. (1961) have reported
identical complications after deep hypothermia. Perhaps some of
these complications depend on an alteration of the brain which
probably takes place during extremely deep cooling. However it
must be remembered that the reported complications have been
observed in cases of cardiac surgery with extracorporeal circulation
and circulatory arrest, whose importance must be not overlooked.

Summary

The authors describe the neurological and psychiatric changes
provoked by therapeutic or accidental hypothermia in patients who

were in a condition which can be regarded as hypothermia without premedication.

Firstly, the changes in consciousness, in speech, in movements and in reflexes were examined. Then the authors studied the influence of hypothermia on those neurological symptoms which develop after the induction of the hypothermic state.

They stress the practical importance of the following observations:

a) Consciousness is preserved with temperatures as low as 30° — 31° C.

b) Hypothermia alone does not induce the appearance of pathological reflexes (Babinski), but it can increase the deep reflexes. However, the development of increased deep reflexes (clonus etc.) is always bilateral and symmetrical.

c) The pupillary light reflex is very sluggish in hypothermia. The pupillary reaction can become so slow as to appear to be absent.

d) Neurological symptoms present before the induction of hypothermia remain unchanged during and after the hypothermic state. However, it must be stressed that in the hypothermic patient the neurological symptoms are more difficult to elicit than in the normothermic.

e) When moderate hypothermia does not produce by itself any lesions whatsoever of the central nervous system which can be proved clinically.

Zusammenfassung

Die Autoren beschreiben die neurologischen und psychischen Veränderungen, die durch Hypothermie (therapeutische oder akzidentelle) bei Patienten hervorgerufen werden, die sich in einem Zustand befinden, der als eine Art Hypothermie ohne Praemedikation bezeichnet werden kann.

Zunächst werden die Veränderungen der Bewußtseinslage, der Sprache, der Motilität und der Reflexe untersucht. Anschließend besprechen die Autoren den Einfluß der Hypothermie auf neurologische Symptome, die wahrscheinlich schon vor der Hypothermie vorhanden waren.

Sie betonen die praktische Bedeutung der folgenden Beobachtungen:

a) Bis 30° — 31° C Körpertemperatur ist das Bewußtsein erhalten.

b) Die Hypothermie als solche verursacht kein Auftreten pathologischer Reflexe (Babinski), kann aber eine Steigerung der tiefen Reflexe hervorrufen; immer sind aber die Erscheinungen der tiefen Hyperreflexie (Kloni usw.) bilateral symmetrisch ausgeprägt.

c) Die Pupillenreaktion auf Licht wird in Hypothermie verlangsamt; die Pupillenreaktion kann so langsam werden, daß sie zu fehlen scheint.

d) Eine schon vorher vorhandene neurologische Symptomatik bleibt während und nach mäßiger Hypothermie unverändert. Es muß allerdings betont werden, daß es bei Patienten in Hypothermie schwieriger ist, die neurologischen Symptome nachzuweisen als in Normothermie.

e) Die gemäßigte Hypothermie erzeugt von sich aus keinerlei Läsionen des zentralen Nervensystems, die klinisch nachgewiesen werden können.

Résumé

Les auteurs décrivent les modifications neurologiques et psychiques
causées par l'hypothermie (thérapeutique ou accidentelle) chez des patients
qui se trouvent dans un état pouvant être qualifié d'hypothermie sans pré-
médication.

Ils décrivent d'abord les modifications de l'état de conscience, de la langue,
de la motilité et des réflexes. Ensuite les auteurs décrivent l'influence de
l'hypothermie sur les signes neurologiques préexistants.

Ils insistent sur la signification pratique des observations suivantes:

a) La conscience persiste jusqu'à la température de 30°—31°.

b) L'hypothermie ne provoque pas l'apparition de réflexes pathologiques
(Babinski), mais elle donne lieu à une hyperréflexie profonde (clonus)
toujours de symétrie bilatérale.

c) La réaction pupillaire à la lumière est ralentie; elle peut être ralentie
au point de sembler faire défaut.

d) Une symptomatologie neurologique préexistante reste inchangée au
cours et après une hypothermie modérée. Il faut cependant noter qu'il est
moins aisé de prouver les symptômes neurologiques en hypothermie qu'en
normothermie.

e) L'hypothermie modérée ne produit pas d'elle-même des lésions quel-
conque du système nerveux central qui peuvent être trouvées cliniquement.

Riassunto

Gli autori descrivono le modificazioni neurologiche e psichiche provo-
cate dalla ipotermia (terapeutica o accidentale) in pazienti che si trovino in
condizioni tali da poter essere considerati in stato di ipotermia senza premedi-
cazione.

Dopo avere esaminato le modificazioni della coscienza, della parola
e della motilità gli autori esaminano le modificazioni dei riflessi e studiano
l'influenza della ipotermia sui sintomi neurologici eventualmente presenti
prima della iduzione dello stato ipotermico.

Si segnala l'interesse pratico delle seguenti osservazioni:

a) Fino a 30°—31° C di temperatura corporea la coscienza é conservata.

b) La ipotermia di per se non provoca la comparsa di riflessi patologici
(Babinski), ma può provocare un 'accentuazione dei riflessi profondi: tuttavia
le manifestazioni di iperreflessia profonda (comparsa di cloni, etc.) sono sempre bilaterali e simmetriche.

c) Il riflesso pupillare alla luce in ipotermia é molto torpido: la contrazione
pupillare é così lenta da sembrare assente.

d) La sintomatologia neurologica eventualmente presente prima della
induzione della ipotermia moderata rimane immodificata durante e dopo
stato ipotermico. Si deve tuttavia segnalare che nel paziente in stato ipotermico i sintomi neurologici sono più difficili da evidenziare che in normotermia.

e) L'ipotermia moderata di per se non produce lesioni del sistema nervoso
centrale dimostrabili clinicamente.

Resumen

Los autores describen las alteraciones neurologicas y psiquiatricas causadas por la hipotermia (terapeutica o accidental) en pacientes que se encuen-
tran en un estado que puede llamarse hipotermia sin premedicacion.

Se revisa en primer lugar las alteraciones de conciencia, del habla, de la motilidad y de los reflejos. Luego los autores comentan la influencia de la hipotermia sobre los sintomas neurologicos que existian probablemente ya antes de la hipotermia.

Ellos insisten sobre la importancia practica de las siguientes observaciones:

a) hasta temperaturas corporales de 30—31⁰ C se conserva la conciencia.

b) la hipotermia en si no provoca la presentacion de reflejos patologicos (Babinski), pero puede causar una acentuacion de los reflejos profundos; estos fenomenos de hiperreflexia profunda (clonos etc.) se demuestran siempre bilaterales.

c) las reacciones pupilares a la luz se retardan en la hipotermia; pueden ser tan lentas, que parecen faltar.

d) una sintomatologia neurologica ya existente se conserva inalterada daurante la hipotermia. Verdad es, que en pacientes bajo hipotermia resulta mucho mas dificil la comprobacion de sintomas neurologicos que bajo normotermia.

e) la hipotermia moderada no produce por sí lesiones del sistema nervioso central que pueden ser provadas clínicamente.

References

Alexander, L.: Treatment of shock from prolonged exposure to cold, especially in water. Report n° 250, U.S. Dept. of Commerce. 1945. — *Bergouignan, M., F. Fontan, M. Trarieux,* and *J. Julien:* Syndromes choréiformes de l'enfant au décours d'intervention cardio-chirurgicales sous hypothermie profonde. Rev. Neurol. *105* (1961), 48—60. — *Bourneville:* Abaissement de la température rectale chez un homme exposé au froid extérieur. Gaz. Höp. *45* (1872), 32—33. — *Britton, S. W.:* Effects of lowering the temperature of homoiothermic animals. Quart. J. Exp. Physiol. *13* (1923), 55—68. — *Callaghan, J. C., D. A. Mac Queen, J. W. Scott,* and *W. G. Bigelow:* Cerebral effects of experimental hypothermia. Arch. Surg. *68* (1954), 208—215. — *Capron, P.:* A propos d'un cas d'hypothermie accidentelle a 24° C, chez l'adulte, suivi de guérison. Bull. Soc. Med. Hop. *74* (1958), 587—591. — *de Grailly, R., H. Leger, J. Kermarec, J. Ph. Leuret, M. Lasserre,* and *E. Cohadon:* Nouvelle observation d'hypothermie profonde accidentelle. Bull. Soc. Med. Hop. *74* (1959), 143—147. — *Delay, J., P. Deniker, D. Ginestet, J. Verdeaux,* and *N. R. Traubendberg:* Effects neuropsychiques des interventions avec arret circulatoire prolongé en hypothermie profonde. (Bilan neuropsychiatrique, psychometrique et electroencephalographique.) Presse Med. *69* (1961), 2539—2542. — *Emslie-Smith, D.:* Accidental hypothermia. A common condition with a pathognomonic electro-cardiogram. Lancet *11* (1958), 492—495. — *Fay, T.:* Observations on prolonged human refrigeration. N. Y. State J. Med. *40* (1940), 1351—1354. — *Fay, T.:* Observations on generalized refrigeration in cases of severe cerebral trauma. Res. Publ. Ass. Nerv. Ment. Dis. *25* (1945), 611—619. — *Fay, T.,* and *G. W. Smith:* Observations on reflex responses during prolonged periods of human refrigeration. Arch. Neurol. Psychiat. *45* (1941), 215—222. — *Gerasimenko, N. I.,* quoted by *Karpovich, O. A.,* in: The problem of acute hypothermia, ed. by *Starkov, P. M.:* 319 p. London: Pergamon Press. 1960. — *Gerster, J. C. A., C. H. Kossman, C. Reich, A. Bernhard, J. Geiger, T. K. Davis, H. R. Kenyon, J. F. Dixon, F. Huber, R. M. Paltauf,* and *W. L. Whitemore:* General cryotherapy: a symposium. Bull. N. Y. Acad. Med. *16* (1940), 312—348. — *Haterius, H. O.,* and *A. B. Hegnauer:* Consciousness and reflex potentialities of dogs during immersion hypothermia. Fed. Proc. *8* (1949), 69—70. — *Justin-Besançon, L., H. Pequignot,* and *J. P. Etienne:* a) Les hypothermies acciden-telles profondes chez l'adulte. Etude clinique et biologique. Sem. Hôp. *34* (1958), 69—84. b) Un cas de réfreigération à 23.5°C suivi de guérison. Sem. Hôp. *34* (1958), 84—90. — *Justin-Besançon, L., H. Pequignot, J. P. Etienne, P. Mauvais-Jarvis,* and *J. P. Gay:* a) Les hypothermies accidentelles. Schweiz. Med. Wschr. *90* (1960), 940—945. b) Nouvelle observation d'hypothermie accidentelle de l'adulte. Rev. Méd. Franc. (1960), 777—791. — *Laufmann, H.:* Profound accidental hypothermia. J.A.M.A. *147* (1951), 1201—1210. — *Lazorthes, G.,* and *L. Campan:* Hypothermia in the treatment of cranio — cerebral traumatism. J. Neurosurg. *15* (1958), 162—167. — *Mares, J.,* and *B. Hellich,* quoted by *Talbott, J. H.,* and *K. J. Tillotson.* 1941. — *Meyer, J. S.,* and *J. Hunter:* Effects of hypothermia on local blood flow and metabolism during cerebral ischemia and hypoxia. J. Neurosurg. *14* (1957), 210—227. — *Pestel, M., J. Tremolieres, L. Carre,* and *J. Cros:* Hypothermie accidentelle a 23.5°C réversible chez un éthylique. Etude physiopathologique du méca-nisme de réchauffement. Press. Med. *69* (1961), 803—805. — *Peter, M.:* Des températures basses excessives. Gaz. hebd. Méd. Chir. *9* (1872), 499—511. — *Reincke, J. J.:* Beobachtungen über die Körpertemperatur Be-trunkener. Dtsch. Arch. Klin. Med. *16* (1875), 12—19. — *Reinhard, C.:* Zur Kasuistik der niedrigsten subnormalen Körpertemperaturen bei Menschen, nebst einigen Bemerkungen über Wärmeregulierung. Berl. Klin. Wschr. *21* (1884), 540—547. — *Rees, J. R.:* Accidental hypothermia. Lancet *1* (1958), 556—559. — *Rosenstiel, M.:* Recherches allemandes sur l'hypothermie provoquée chez les animaux et chez les hommes. Press. Med. *1946,* 257—258. — *Simpson, S.,* 1902 quoted by *Simpson, S.,* and *P. T. Herring.* 1905. — *Simpson, S.,* and *P. T. Herring:* The effect of cold narcosis on reflex action in warm-blooded animals. J. Physiol. *32* (1905), 305—311. — *Spradley, J. B.,* and *M. Marin Foucher:* Hypothermia (a new treatment of psychiatric dis-orders). Dis. nerv. Syst. *10* (1949), 235—238. — *Starkov, P. M.:* The problem of acute hypothermia, 319 p. London: Pergamon Press. 1960. — *Streit, K.:* Zur Therapie der allgemeinen Unterkühlung. Vjschr. Schweiz. Sanit. Off. *32* (1955), n° 4. — *Talbott, J. H.:* The physiologic and therapeutic effects of hypothermia. New Engl. J. Med. *224* (1941), 281—288. — *Talbott, J. H.:* Cold exposure: pathologic effects. In "Medical Physics", vol. 1, ed. by *O. Glasser,* 1744 p. Chicago: Year Book Publ. 1944. — *Talbott, J. H.,* and *K. J. Tillotson:* The effect of cold on mental disorders. A study of the patients suffering from schizophrenia and treated with hypothermia. Dis. nerv. Syst. *2* (1941), 116—126. — *Wayburn, E.:* Immersion hypothermia. Arch. Int. med. *79* (1947), 77—91. — *Walther,* 1862 quoted by *Simpson, S.,* and *P. T. Her-ring.* 1905.

Clinica Neurochirurgica — Università degli Studi — Milano (Italy)
Service d'Eléctroencéphalographie — Hôpital Neurologique — Lyon (France)

Electroencephalographic Modifications Induced by Moderate and Deep Hypothermia in Man

By

C. A. Pagni and J. Courjon

With 6 Figures

The EEG modifications provoked by moderate hypothermia (down to 28° C) differ considerably from those observed in deep hypothermia (lower than 28° C).

1. Moderate Hypothermia

The EEG modifications induced in man by moderate hypothermia are very mild.

Hale and *Moraca* (1958) state that as the temperature falls the voltage drops. According to *Scott* (1958) at about 30° C the voltage is about half that at normal temperature and some delta waves appear but they usually are not prominent.

Werman and *Baronofsky* (1958), *Kubicki* and *Just* (1959), *Pearcy* and *Virtue* (1959), *Kubicki* et al. (1960) report that down to 28°—29° C generally there are no clear modifications of the EEG; sometimes there is a very mild slowing of EEG activity. *Van Buren* et al. (1960) observed that moderate hypothermia in anaesthetized patients, induced little change in the general pattern of the electrocorticographic activity.

Our observations performed in 20 cases of moderate hypothermia (down to 28° C) with electroencephalographic and/or electrodurographic, and/or electrocorticographic records, agree with the data of the literature.

The EEG aspects observed between 36° and 28° C differ only slightly from those seen under normothermic conditions.

Four types of recordings may be distinguished:

a) recordings that do not differ from those of normothermia;

b) recordings that show a very moderate fall in amplitude of cortical activity with or without changes of frequency;

c) recordings characterized by a slight decrease in the frequency;

d) recordings with special variations. In cases in which a very rapid cooling by veno-venous shunt was obtained, theta activity of moderate high voltage appeared during cooling from 36° to 30° C. After the fall of temperature ceased theta activity disappeared and the EEG recovered the pattern which it showed before the cooling.

Our experience agrees with the observations of the previously reported authors and with the results of experiments on animals. Also in animals moderate hypothermia induces only a moderate fall in the amplitude of electrocorticographic activity (*ten Cate* et al., 1949; *Kayser* et al., 1951; *Scott* et al., 1953; *Koella* and *Ballin*, 1954; *de Castro*, 1956; *Jouvet* et al., 1956; *Bok* and *Shadé*, 1957; *Bryce-Smith* et al., 1960). During cooling from 36° to 30° C a moderate increase of amplitude of EEG was observed in animals (*ten Cate* et al., 1949; *Bok* and *Shadé*, 1957; *Suda* et al., 1957).

In man during moderate hypothermia we never observed spontaneous convulsive activity. On the contrary *Weinstein* et al. (1961) report cortical convulsive spontaneous activity in animal experiments between 34° and 28° C.

Many authors have reported an increase of excitability of the central nervous system with moderate cooling in animals. *Barron* and *Matthews* (1939) report augmentation of dorsal-root reflexes at 31° C. *Suda* et al. (1956) report an increase in the cerebellar and cortical evoked potentials and *Brooks* et al. (1955), *Grundfest* (1941), *Suda* et al. (1957) report an increase in magnitude of the spinal reflex potentials at about 35°—32° C in cats. *Noell* et al. (1952), *Noell* and *Briller* (1953) reported a lowering of threshold for electrical after-discharge below 35°—30° C in rabbits, and *Chardon* and *Bonnet* (1958) reported similar results.

Also drug sensitivity of the central nervous system is increased in moderate hypothermia in animals according to *Noell* and *Briller* (1953). On the contrary *Owens* (1958) observed an increase of the threshold for the electrical after-discharge at 28°—26° C.

In an attempt to make a contribution to the question of the electrical excitability of the cerebral cortex during moderate hypothermia in man, we have performed 18 cortical electrical stimulations in three patients during hypothermia. The patients were premedicated with Largactil, Demerol, Scopolamine; anaesthesia was induced with Pentothal, and maintained with Fluothane, Oxygen, N_2O. Electrical stimulations were performed in the Rolandic and parietal region with chlorurated silver electrodes, spaced 2 mm. apart, using 5 msec. unidirectional square wave pulses, 60 per sec., at 5—25 V.

In our cases we have obtained no electrical after-discharge.

Our results agree with the experience of *van Buren* et al. (1960) who in patients with body temperatures between 28.6°—30.4° C obtained only one after-discharge in 140 stimulations.

These contradictory results between animal and clinical experiences in moderate hypothermia are difficult to explain. It may be, as *van Buren* et al. (1960) pointed out, that different anaesthesia and eventually anoxia play a big role in modification of excitability of the central nervous system in some of the reported experiences.

2. Deep Hypothermia

Below 28° C the electroencephalographic modifications induced by hypothermia are very pronounced.

We report the results of an electroencephalographic study on 75 cases of patients affected by cardiovascular diseases and submitted to operation under deep hypothermia (down to 7° C) with extracorporeal circulation.

The electroencephalographic changes induced by progressive lowering of body temperature and by the following rewarming may be described according to a fairly constant scheme.

A) Cooling Period

a) Phase of Progressive Slowing and Disorganization of the EEG

Below 28°—25° C there is a progressive slowing of the cortical electrical activity. After a phase of theta activity a disorganized, high voltage delta activity appears (Fig. 1 *B*).

The rate of cooling has a direct bearing on the velocity of slowing and of disorganization of the EEG. If the cooling is slow, the theta activity persists for a very long time. With very rapid cooling the delta activity appears earlier: the stages of progressive slowing of the EEG are shortened.

It must be pointed out also that the age of the patient has a direct bearing on the rate of slowing of the EEG: in the young the slowing is swift and more remarkable than in the adult. In some cases a noticeable slowing of the EEG can be observed at very high body temperature when extracorporeal circulation has been started, as has been observed also by *Trede* et al. (1959).

b) Phase of Paroxysmal Cortical Activity

Below a body temperature of 20°—15° C high voltage slow spikes and spike and wave complexes are recorded.

Generally the slow spike complexes are bilaterally synchronous (Fig. 2), but sometimes they can appear, at the beginning, only over one hemisphere and over the temporal region (Fig. 1 *B*).

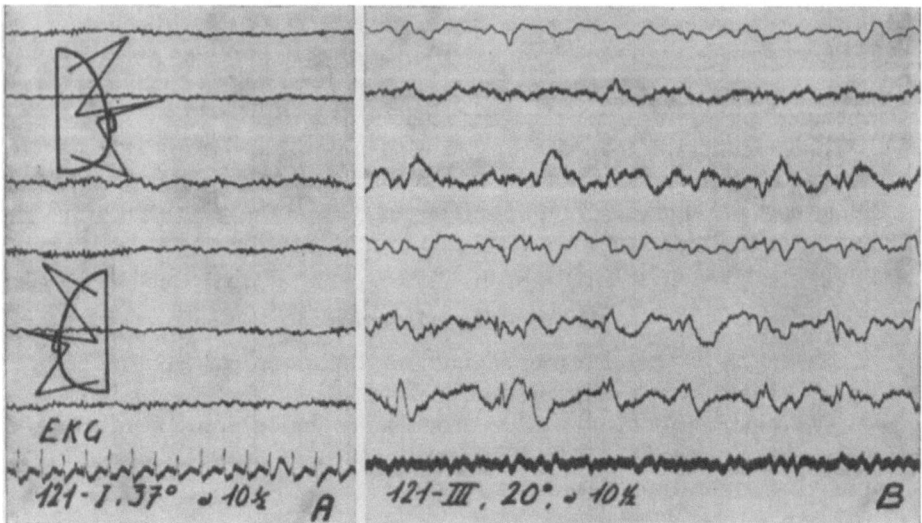

Fig. 1. Channels 1—6: scalp EEG; Channel 7: EKG; Case 121 aged 10 years and 6 months. *A* Before cooling; *B* Diffuse disorganization and slowing of the EEG at 20° C of oesophageal temperature. Note slow spike and waves complexes in the left temporo-occipital leads

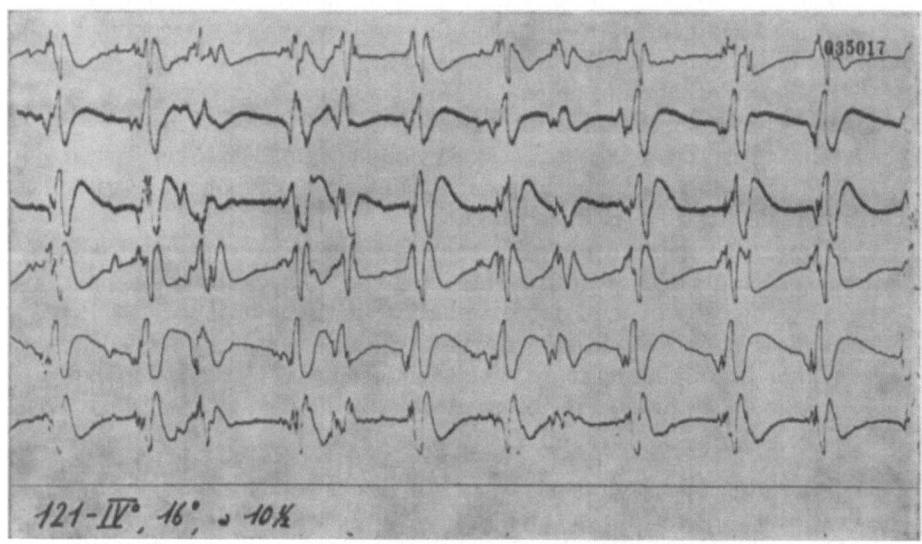

Fig. 2. Case 121. Derivation, calibration as in Fig. 1. The EEG pattern at 16°C of oesophageal temperature is characterized by very high voltage, bilaterally synchronous spike and wave complexes

At the beginning the tracings show bursts of these paroxysmal complexes associated and intermixed with delta activity.

The slow spike-wave complexes are recorded generally only in young people under 15 years. These spike complexes are not recorded in adults.

With progressive lowering of body temperature the spikes of the paroxysmal complexes become progressively degraded and deformed. The tracings show paroxysmal bursts of slow waves of high voltage. This pattern is typical of adults in whom spike discharges are seldom recorded.

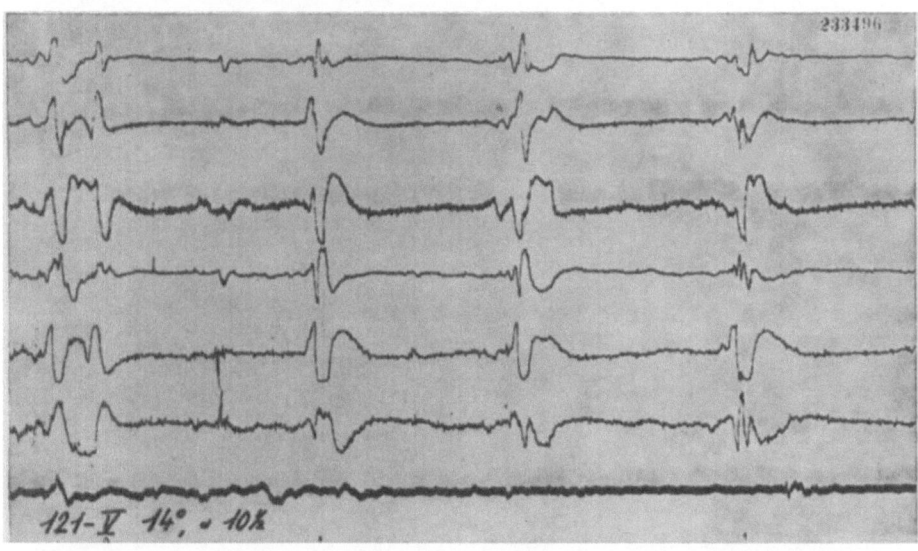

Fig. 3. Case 121. Derivation, calibration as in Fig. 1. At an oesophageal tempera-ture of 14° C the bursts of spike and wave complexes are separated by phases of suppression of the tracing. The paroxysmal bursts have a periodic recurrence

c) *Phase of the "Suppression Bursts" Activity*

With a further lowering of the body temperature the bursts of spike-and-wave complexes are separated by pauses of several seconds during which the base-line remains nearly flat. With the occurrence of these short periods of "black out" the tracings show a pattern of "suppression bursts" (Fig. 3). These changes may be observed at the beginning only over one hemisphere.

In this phase the tracings often show typical periodic recurrence of the paroxysmal complexes; sometimes the pattern is identical with the "periodic" tracings of subacute sclerosing leucoencephalopathy (Fig. 4). It is characterized by the monotonous recurrence, on a given derivation, of a paroxysmal complex of constant shape.

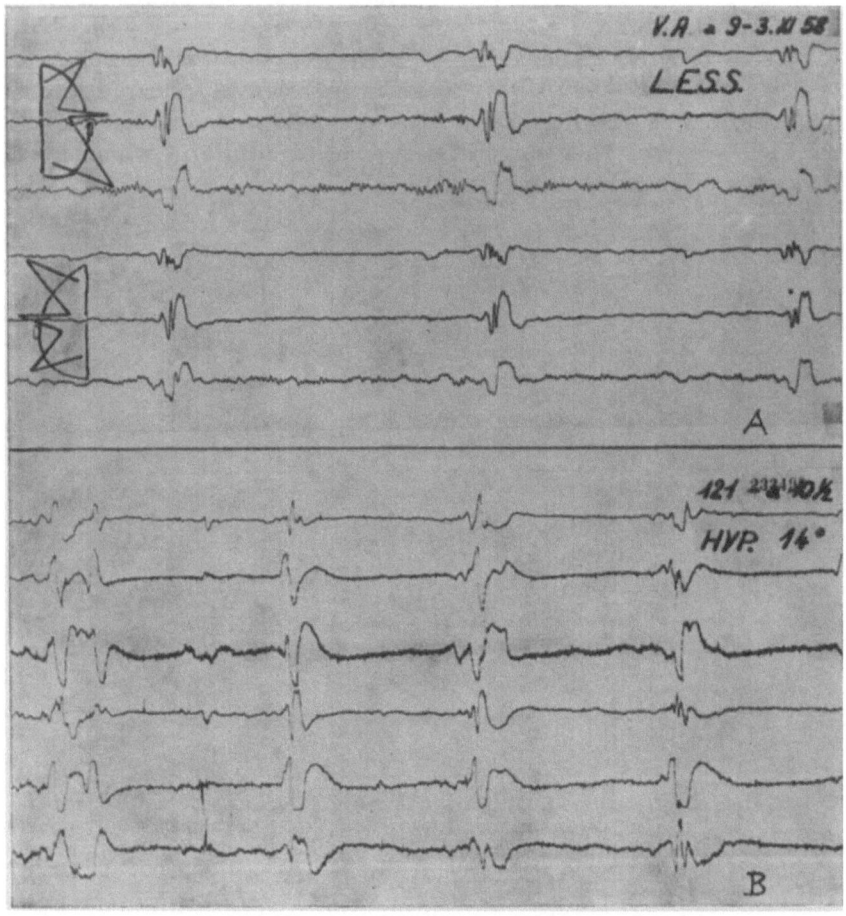

Fig. 4. In the upper part of the figure (*A*) is reproduced a specimen of the tracing of a Sclerosing Subacute Leucoencephalopathy (LESS). In the lower part (*B*) the E G G of a patient during deep hypothermia at an oesophageal temperature of 14° C is shown. Note in both tracings the periodic monotonous recurrence of paroxysmal complexes of constant shape

At about 10° C of body temperature the periods of "black out" are very long and the paroxysmal complexes recur periodically every 30—60 seconds.

At a very low temperature the tracings are sometimes very similar to the tracings of a premature baby.

d) *Phase of the Flat Recording (Tracé Nul)*

At a very low temperature the spontaneous cortical activity disappears and the tracings are flat and display only some very low amplitude waves.

Rapid cooling results in an earlier loss of amplitude and near isoelectric tracings appear at higher temperature than in patients cooled more slowly.

But it must be remembered that neither the rate of cooling nor the age of the patients explain wholly the earlier or later loss of electrical activity. In some cases the loss of electrical activity is complete at a body temperature of 17° C; in other cases at 7° C the spontaneous electrical activity is still present. Some unknown individual factor has certainly a direct bearing on this point.

B) Rewarming Period

e) *Phase of Permanent Microvoltage*

Immediately after the beginning of rewarming the paroxismal complexes, if still present, disappear: the tracings are near isoelectric (Fig. 5A, B) or characterized by a very low voltage, slow activity.

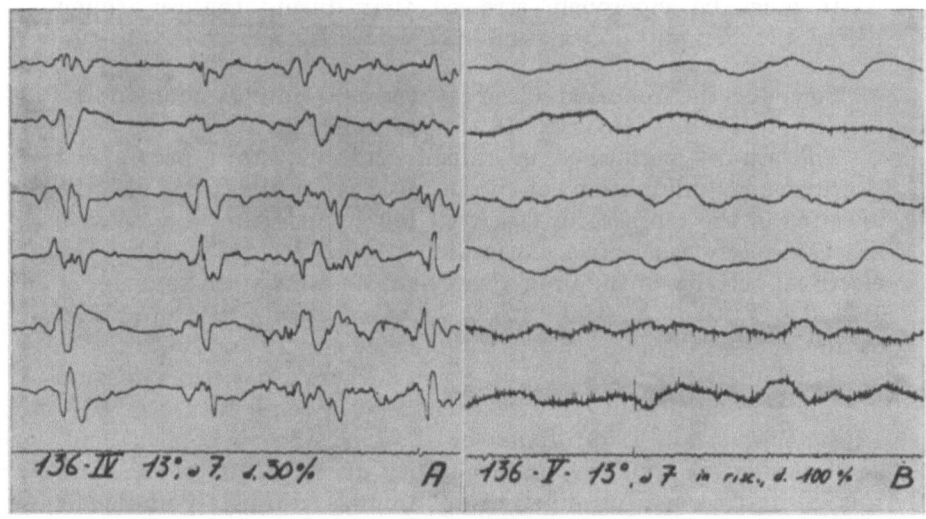

Fig. 5. Immediately after the beginning of recirculation of warm blood (B) the paroxysmal complexes disappear, even if the body temperature has not yet changed

f) Phase of Bursts at 8 Cycle per Second

Brain activity reappears on warming at a body temperature higher than the temperature at which the electrical activity disappeared on cooling.

At 30° C of body temperature, particularly in adults, bursts of sinusoidal rhythmical waves at 8 cycle per second, were observed, lasting some seconds and of an amplitude varying from 20 to 60 microvolts.

These bursts, localized over the frontal or fronto-central areas are indistinguishable from the spindle bursts observed in certain cases of coma having an EEG pattern like "cerveau isolé" (personal observations).

The spindles at 8 cycle per second are sometimes intermixed with varying degrees of widespread delta and theta activity.

This phase was observed only in a few cases.

g) Phase of Restoration of Normal Frequencies

At body temperature of 30°—32° C, generally, some low voltage, irregular, sporadic, very slow delta activity reappears. Thereafter in parieto-occipital areas theta activity appears, always intermixed with delta activity. Subsequently more rapid waves also reappear; at 37° C, if there have not been cardiac complications, the tracings display a near normal pattern.

It must be vigorously stressed that during the rewarming period the periodic paroxysmal complexes are not observed.

Some of the reported observations are quite similar to the results of electrocorticographic studies in animals.

The studies performed in animals demonstrate a progressive slowing and diminution of brain-wave amplitude due to the lowering of the temperature; at very low temperature the tracings are essentially isoelectric. According to the various authors the electrical activity of the brain disappears at a body temperature of 16°—24° C (ten Cate et al., 1949; Chatfield et al., 1951; Gänshirt et al., 1954; Cazzullo, 1956; McQueen et al., 1959; Bryce-Smith et al., 1960; Lourie et al., 1960). Some authors report that in some instances brain activity is still present at a temperature of 8°—12° C (Scott et al., 1953; Jouvet et al., 1956; Lourie et al., 1960). A persisting spontaneous brain activity at very low temperature was also observed in hibernating animals during spontaneous or induced hibernation (Lyman et Chatfield, 1953; Kayser et al., 1951).

The differences in temperatures at which the electrical activity of the brain disappears are due, perhaps, to different experimental conditions.

For instance, according to *Lourie* et al. (1960) in dogs rapid cooling results in earlier loss of amplitude and near isoelectric tracings would appear at higher temperatures than in dogs cooled more slowly. According to *Bryce-Smith* et al. (1960) the isoelectric tracing appears at a higher body temperature in animals anaesthetized with pentobarbitone than in those anaesthetized with ether.

In man we have observed that brain activity sometimes disappears even at 17° C of body temperature, but in some cases brain activity persists at a temperature as low as 7° C.

We believe that even in the human the rate of cooling has a direct bearing on the earlier or later loss of electrical brain activity. Nevertheless this is not a sufficient explanation: individual factors which escape us and the characteristics of the extracorporeal circulation (*Arfel*, 1962) are certainly important.

In animal experiments a tendency to spike activity during deep hypothermia has been reported by many authors.

Jouvet et al. (1956) report in curarized cats bilateral spikes at 17° C and seizures at lower temperatures.

Chardon et *Bonnet* (1959) described spikes and electrical seizures during hyperventilation in hypothermic dogs, and *McQueen* et al. (1957) state that spike activity is more prominent during O_2 breathing.

Malmejac et *Chardon* (1959) report that the intravenous administration of adrenaline at 20° C provokes convulsive discharges.

Weinstein et al. (1961) observed spontaneous electroclinical seizures in hypothermic dogs.

Lourie et al. (1960), *de Rougemont* et al. (1962) state that spike activity begins at 26°—28° C during selective cerebral hypothermia in dogs.

In man, during cooling, paroxysmal spike activity appears generally at body temperatures of 20°—15° C, and as we have previously stated only in subjects under fifteen years of age (Fig. 6).

According to our experience it is impossible to find a direct correlation between body temperature and the characteristics of the electroencephalographic phases. Also, if generally the slowing of the EEG begins at 25°C and the spike activity between 20° and 15°C, in different subjects of the same age at the same body temperature the paroxysmal spike complexes may be more or less slow, frequent and prominent. It is not yet possible to give to these differences a particular prognostic significance.

We will now examine the effects of circulatory arrest on the electroencephalographic activity of hypothermic patients. Moreover

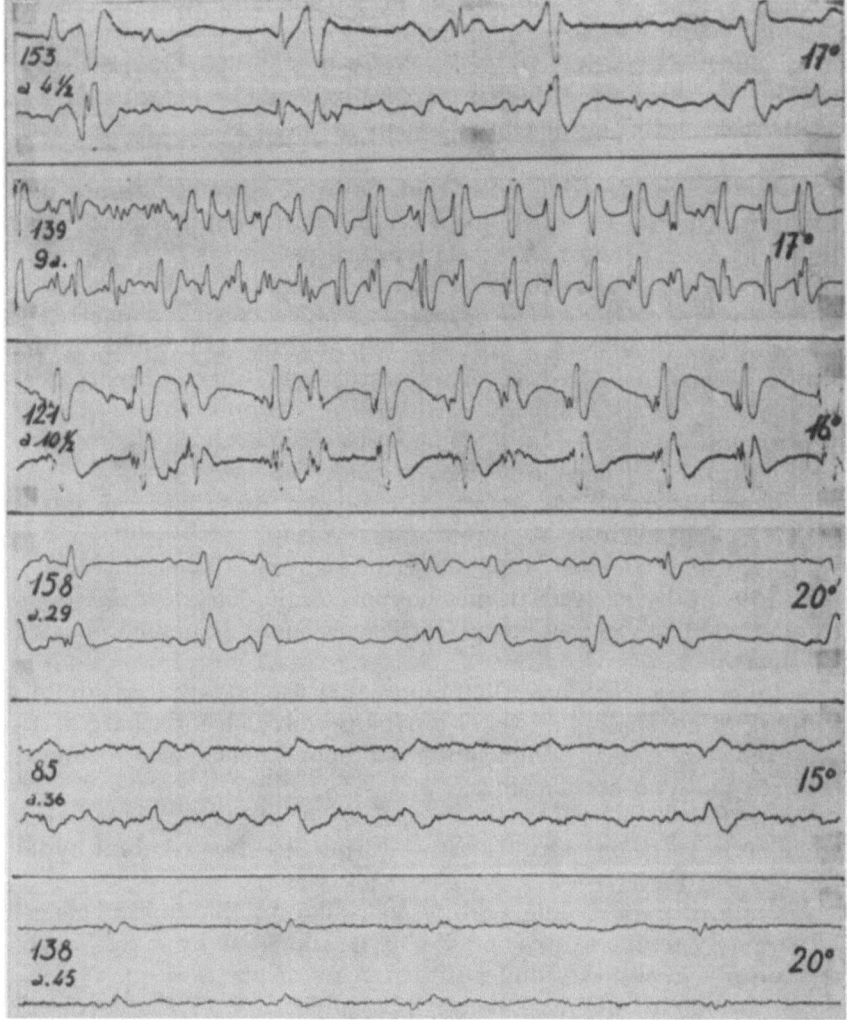

Fig. 6. Different EEG pattern at body temperature of 15°—20° C in patients of different age. Note that spike activity is observed only in young people (cases 153, 139, 121, respectively aged 4¹/₂, 9, 10¹/₂) and not in adults (cases 158, 85, 138, respectively aged 29, 36, 45)

we will examine how and how long after the re-establishment of blood circulation the electroencephalographic activity is recovered, and if from these electroencephalographic data we can obtain useful prognostic indications.

According to our experience complete circulatory arrest provokes the complete suppression of every electroencephalographic activity in 30—60 seconds: this period is the so-called *"survival period"* of the tracings. Our data do not agree with those of other authors who give electroencephalographic survival periods of even 120 seconds or more in moderate or deep hypothermia at oesophageal temperature of 15° C (*Clutton Brock*, 1959; *Arfel* et al., 1963). According to our experience there is not a strict relation between oesophageal temperature and survival time of the EEG. We also believe that the duration of the "survival period" of the tracings in deep hypothermia has no prognostic importance, because it is not related to the recovery of cerebral activity.

In ten cases out of our seventy five, complete circulatory arrest was prolonged for periods of 6 to 50 minutes at oesophageal temperatures of 15°—7° C: this had no disadvantageous consequence for the recovery of the electroencephalographic activity and of the patient. Low temperatures allow therefore particularly long circulatory arrests without any cerebral damage.

After circulatory arrest the interval between the moment in which the circulation is resumed and the moment in which the electroencephalographic activity reappears is the *"latence de ré-cupération"*. The duration of this interval is not dependent, according to us, on the duration of the circulatory arrest, but it depends only on the deepness of hypothermia and on the speed of rewarming.

In fact, as we have seen before, during the rewarming period it is necessary to reach 30° C body temperature for electroencephalographic activity to reappear. Short periods of re-circulation, of 2—3 minutes, during long circulatory arrests do not appear to facilitate faster electroencephalographic recovery.

In our experience then, the *"latence de récupération"* which is a function of the rewarming velocity, cannot give any prognostic indication.

Also the measurement of the *"recovery time"*, that is the time between the re-establishment of circulation and the re-appearance of a normal tracing does not give sure prognostic indications. Experience has demonstrated that if excessively long "recovery time" with persistence of very slow waves of high voltage may indicate a certain cerebral damage, a perfect recovery without neurological consequences is nevertheless possible.

On the contrary we think it is very important to study the morphological characteristics of the electroencephalographic trac-

ings at the time the electrical activity reappears. The appearance
of bursts of spikes and spike-and-waves during the rewarming of
the patient has a great prognostic importance: they demonstrate a
certain cerebral damage and mean that epileptic seizures must
be expected in they following hours.

In fact as we have said before, while describing the phases of
the rewarming period, during rewarming, paroxysmal spike complexes are not observed, the contrary of what happens during
cooling. If irritative abnormalities appear they can be followed by
generalized myoclonus and seizures.

Epileptic complications after deep hypothermia are particularly
dangerous: 5 cases of 7 in whom the were observed, died.

We have observed electrical seizures localized to one cerebral
hemisphere in two cases of patients who died: perhaps a gas
embolus was the cause of these seizures.

Summary

The authors describe the changes in the cerebral electrical activity induced by moderate and deep hypothermia. The changes
with moderate hypothermia (not below 28° C) are very slight.

By contrast, deep hypothermia (below 28° C) provokes very obvious changes in the E. E. G. After an initial phase, there is a progressive delta disorganisation of the tracing until there is paroxysmal activity consisting of slow spike and wave complexes which
recur periodically. With further lowering of the body temperature
the paroxysmal activity decreases progressively and finally disappears. If the body temperature is lowered to 14° C the E. E. G. tracing is depressed and virtually reduced to an iso-electric line.

Rewarming of the patient results in a progressive restoration of
the normal frequencies: however, it must be especially stressed that,
during rewarming, the E. E. G. activity is only resumed at a fairly
high temperature and it does pass through a phase of periodic paroxysmal activity. The authors discuss the prognostic value of the
E. E. G. record obtained in deep hypothermia: it appears that the
appearance of electrographic epileptic features during rewarming
indicates damage to the brain.

Zusammenfassung

Die Autoren beschreiben die Veränderungen der zerebralen elektrischen
Aktivität, die durch mäßige und tiefe Hypothermie hervorgerufen werden.
Die Veränderungen durch mäßige Hypothermie sind ziemlich geringfügig.

Tiefe Hypothermie (unter 28° C) verursacht dagegen deutlichere Veränderungen des EEG. Nach einer anfänglichen, fortschreitenden Phase unregel-

mäßiger Delta-Aktivität folgen paroxysmale Entladungen, die aus langsamen Spike-Wave-Mustern bestehen und sich periodisch wiederholen. Mit weiterem Absinken der Körpertemperatur nehmen diese paroxysmalen Gruppen ab und verschwinden schließlich. Wenn die Körpertemperatur auf 14° C abgesunken ist, entspricht die EEG-Kurve praktisch einer isoelektrischen Linie.

Die Wiedererwärmung des Patienten bewirkt ein zunehmendes Wiederauftreten normaler Frequenzen: vor allem muß betont werden, daß während der Erwärmung die EEG-Aktivität erst bei höherer Temperatur wieder einsetzt, und ohne daß die Phase periodischer paroxysmaler Aktivität wieder durchlaufen wird.

Die Autoren diskutieren den prognostischen Wert des EEG's während der tiefen Hypothermie: Es hat sich gezeigt, daß das Auftreten von Krampfströmen während der Erwärmung das Eintreten eines Hirnschadens anzeigt.

Résumé
Les auteurs décrivent les modifications de l'activité électrique cérébrale induites par l'hypothermie modérée et profonde. Sous hypothermie modérée les modifications sont peu marquées.

L'hypothermie en dessous de 28° fait par contre des modifications plus sensibles de l'EEG. Une première phase d'activité Delta irrégulière est suivie de décharges paroxysmiques formées de „spike waves" lentes et se répétant périodiquement. Ces décharges paroxysmiques diminuent au fur et à mesure que diminue la température, pour disparaître enfin complètement. Quand la température a baissé jusqu'à 14°, l'EGG correspond pratiquement à une ligne isoélectrique.

Le réchauffement du malade produit la réapparition de fréquences normales: il est surtout important de noter que l'activité électroencephalographique ne reprend qu'à une température plus élevée et sans que la phase d'activité paroxysmique périodique ne soit encore une fois parcourue.

Les auteurs discutent de la valeur pronostique de l'EEG dans l'hypothermie profonde: il s'est trouvé que l'apparition d'un tracé paroxysmique au cours du réchauffement dénonce un endommagement cérébral.

Riassunto
Gli autori descrivono le modificazioni indotte dalla ipotermia moderata e profonda sulla attività elettrica cerebrale.

Le modificazioni indotte dalla ipotermia moderata (fino a 28° C) sono molto scarse.

L'ipotermia profonda (sotto 28° C) provaca invece delle modificazioni elettroencefalografiche molto evidenti. Dopo una fase iniziale e progressiva di disorganizzazione delta del tracciato compare una attività parossistica costituita da punte onde lente a ricorrenza periodica. Con l'ulteriore abbassarsi della temperatura coporea queste figure parossistiche si degradano progressivamente fino ad esaurirsi. Quando la temperatura corporea scende al di sotto di 14° C il tracciato EEG é depresso e praticamente ridotto ad una linea isoelettrica.

Il riscaldamento del paziente provoca un progressivo recupero delle frequenze normali: tuttavia si deve segnalare che durante il riscaldamento la attività EEG ricompare solo a temperature molto elevate e senza passare attraverso la fase dei complessi periodici parossistici. Gli autori discutono il valore prognostico dell'EEG registrato in ipotermia profonda: ritengono che la comparsa di figure parossistiche durante il riscaldamento del paziente significhi che si é stabilito un danno cerebrale.

Resumen

Los autores describen las alteraciones de la actividad bioelectrica cerebral causadas por moderada y profunda hipotermia. Las alteraciones por hipotermia moderada son relativamente pocas.

Hipotermia profunda (debajo de 28°) al contrario causa acentuadas modificationes en el EEG. Despues de una primera y progresiva fase de actividad delta irregular siguen descargas paroxisticas, que consisten de lentos grupos con espigas y ondas en repeticion periodica. Con el siguiente descenso de la temperatura corporal se disminuyen estes grupos para desaperecer finalmente. Al llegar la temperatura corporal a los 14° el trazado electroencefalografico corresponde practicamente a una linea isoelectricia.

El recalentamiento del paciente hace la reaparicion de frecuencias normales; hay que insistir en al hecho, que la actividad electroencefalografica reinicia durante el recalentamiento recien con temperaturas mas altas y sin pasar otra vez la fase de actividad periodica paroxistica.

Los autores discuten el valor pronostico del EEG durante la hipotermia profunda; se ha damonstrado, que la presentacion de trazados convulsivos durante el calentamiento señala la aparicion de una lesion cerebral.

References

Arfel, G.: In "L'hypothermie en neurochirurgie", ed. by *Wertheimer, P.,* p. 74—78. Paris: Masson et Cie. 1962. — *Arfel, G., H. Fischgold,* and *J. Weiss:* Le silénce cerebral. In "Problemes de base en électroencéphalographie" ed. by *Fischgold, H., C. Dreyfus-Brisac,* and *Ph. Pruvot,* p. 117—152. Paris: Masson et Cie. 1963. — *Barron, D. H.,* and *B. H. C. Matthews:* Dorsal root reflexes. J. Physiol. *94* (1939), 26—27 P. — *Bok, S. T.,* and *J. P. Shadé:* Hypothermia and cerebral activity. Acta physiol. pharmac. neerl. *6* (1957), 775—784. — *Brooks, C. McC., K. Koizumi,* and *J. L. Malcom:* Effects of changes in temperature on reactions of spinal cord. J. Neurophysiol. *18* (1955), 205—216. — *Bryce-Smith, R., H. G. Epstein,* and *P. Glees:* Physiological studies during hypothermia in monkey. J. Appl. Physiol. *15* (1960), 440—443. — *Buren, J. M. van, F. H. Norris, K. D. Hall,* and *C. Ajmone-Marsan:* The electrographic activity of the cooled human frontal lobe and its response to hypotension. J. Neurosurg. *17* (1960), 905—922. — *Cate, J. ten, G. P. M. Horsten,* and *L. J. Koopman:* The influence of the body temperature on the EEG of the rat. EEG Clin. Neurophysiol. *1* (1949), 231—235. — *Cazzullo, C. L.:* Sistema nervoso e ibernazione artificiale. Rassegna critica e contributo di neurofisiopatologia sperimentale. Riv. Sper. Freniat. *80* (1956), 3—101. — *Chardon, G.,* and *D. Bonnet:* Cortical excitability and induced hypothermia. C.R.Soc. Biol. *153* (1959), 778—780. — *Chardon, G.,* and *D. Bonnet:* Effect of induced hypothermia on excitability of the cortex. C.R. Soc. Biol. *152* (1958), 582—584. — *Chatfield, P. O., C. P. Lyman,* and *D. P. Purpura:* The effect of temperature on the spontaneous and induced electrical activity in the cerebral cortex of the golden hamster. EEG Clin. Neurophysiol. *3* (1951), 225—230. — *Clutton-Brock, J.:* Some details of a technique for hypothermia. Brit. J. Anaesth. *31* (1959), 210—217. — *de Castro, L. R.:* Electroencephalography in dogs during ether anaesthesia: correlation of various electroencephalographic patterns with ether concentrations in arterial blood at normal temperature and at 30 degrees centigrade. Thesis, University of Minnesota. 1956. — *de Rougement, J., J. Descotes, P. George, J. Courjon, M. Piéchon,* et *M. Peysson:* L'hypothermie cérébral sélective.

Données expérimentales. Ann. Chir. *16* (1962), 1403—1412. — *Ganshirt, H., W. Krenkel,* and *W. Zylka:* The electrocorticogram of the cat's brain at temperature between 40° C and 20° C. EEG Clin. Neurophysiol. *6* (1954), 409— 413. — *Grundfest, H.:* The augmentation of the motor root reflexes discharges in the cooled spinal cord of the cat. Am. J. Physiol. *133* (1941), 307 — P. — *Hale, D. E.,* and *P. P. Moraca:* Electrocardiogram and electroencephalogram in elective cardiac arrest J.A.M.A. *166* (1958), 1672—1677. — *Jouvet, M., O. Benoit, J. Courjon,* and *M. Tauche:* The EEG during hypothermia in paralyzed cats. (Cortical and subcortical changes, electrical responses to auditory stimuli and convulsive discharges.) EEG Clin. Neurophysiol. *8* (1956), 708 (Abst.). — *Kayser, C., F. Rohmer* et *G. Hiebel:* L'EEG de l'hibernant. Léthargie et réveil spontanée du spermophile. Essai de reproduction de l'EEG chez le spermophile réveillé et le rat blanc. Rev. Neurol. *84* (1951), 570—578. — *Koella, W. P.,* and *H. M. Ballin:* Influence of environmental and body temperature on electroencephalogram in anaesthetized cat. Arch. Intern. Physiol. *62* (1954), 369—375. — *Kubicki, S.,* und *O. Just:* Das EEG im Verlauf von Herzoperationen mit Kreislaufunterbrechung. Anaesthesist *8* (1959), 1—5. — *Kubicki, S., M. Trede* und *O. Just:* Die Bedeutung des EEG bei Herzoperationen in Hypothermie und bei extrakorporaler Zirkulation. Anaesthesist *9* (1960), 119—123. — *Lyman, C. P.,* and *P. O. Chatfield:* Hibernation and cortical electrical activity in the Woodchuck. Science *117* (1953), 533—534. — *Lourie, H., T. G. Holmes, W. Weinstein, H. G. Schwartz,* and *J. L. O'Leary:* Observations on selective brain cooling in dogs. Arch. Neurol. *3* (1960), 163—176. — *Malméjac, J.,* et *G. Chardon:* Action de l'adrenaline sur l'activité du cortex cérébral à basse température. Bull. Acad. Nat. Med. *143* (1959), 11—12. — *Noell, W. K.,* and *S. A. Briller:* The effect of hypothermia on brain activity. Air Force Sch. Aviat. Med., Randolph Field, Tex., Project n° 21-1202-0003. 1953, 1—33. — *Noell, W. K., S. A. Briller,* and *W. B. Brendel:* Effects of cold exposure on brain activity. Fed. Proc. *11* (1952), 114. — *Owens, G.:* Effects of hypothermia on seizures induced by physical and chemical means. Am. J. Physiol. *193* (1958), 560—562. — *Queen, Mc J. D., R. S. Lichtenstein, G. B. Udvarhelyi,* and *A. A. Earnekian:* Effects of hypothermia upon epileptic discharges. Proc. 1st. Int. Congr. Neurol. Sciences. Bruxelles 1957. Vol. III°, EEG, Clinical Neurophysiol. and Epilepsy, p. 594—599. London: Pergamon Press. 1959. — *Scott, J. W.:* The EEG and hypothermia. Spike and Wave 7 (1958), 6—7. — *Scott, J. W., J. D. McQueen,* and *C. J. Callaghan:* The effect of lowered body temperature on the EEG. EEG Clin. Neurophysiol. *5* (1953), 465 (Abst.). — *Suda, I., K. Koizumi,* and *C. C. McBrooks:* Analysis of effects of hypothermia on central nervous system responses. Am. J. Physiol. *189* (1957), 373—380. — *Suda, I., K. Koizumi,* and *C. C. McBrooks:* Effects of cooling on central nervous system responses. Fed. Proc. *15* (1956), 182. — *Trede, M., S. Kubicki* und *O. Just:* Über EEG-Beobachtungen bei Herzoperationen mit dem extrakorporalen Kreislauf. Anaesthesist *8* (1959), 76—82. — *Weinstein, W., J. H. Kendig, S. Goldring, J. L. O'Leary,* and *H. Lourie:* Hypothermia and electrical activity of cerebral cortex. Arch. Neurol. *4* (1961), 441—448. — *Werman, R.,* and *L. Baronofsky:* EEG changes in open heart surgery. EEG Clin. Neurophysiol. *10* (1958), 205 (Abst.).

II. Hypothermia for Neurosurgical Operations

Clinica Medica — Università degli Studi — Milano (Italy)

Changes in the Blood Clotting Mechanism During Moderate Hypothermia for Neurosurgical Operations

By

R. Locatelli

With 9 Figures

Introduction

The ever increasing number of surgical operations under hypothermia has suggested studies on blood coagulation changes in patients undergoing these operations. Interest was especially centered on surgical procedures for cerebral aneurysm, intra- and post-operative thrombosis and hemorrhage (often lethal) being a common complication.

It is well known that blood coagulation balance is modified to a varying extent by surgery. Hypercoagulability, at times even marked, has been frequently reported [3] [4] [8] in spite of a frequent decrease in the activity of some factors, i. e. of prothrombin. This fact is easily accounted for by an increase in thromboplastinic factors (in a broad sense) and fibrinogen level not counterbalanced by a decreased prothrombin conversion. The pathogenetic causes of these changes are still unexplained. Nevertheless, the increased coagulability may be easily related to the stress exerted on tissues, which are known to be rich in substances with thromboplastin activity.

The other fact we are going to consider, or hypothermia, promotes on the other hand opposite conditions, since temperature decrease is known to exert *in vitro* a clear negative effect on blood coagulatory activity.

Although *in vitro* processes are not exactly superimposable on *in vivo* conditions, we deemed that a parallel could be suggested with observations reported in the literature. In fact, *Montini, Paoletti* and *Piccinini* found during hypothermia a decreased blood coagulability which they interpreted as probably due to a retarded prothrombin conversion caused by a deficiency in the accelerators (Factors V and VII) [5] [6].

These findings, however, were obtained in the experimental animal (rabbits). Moreover, under the experimental conditions employed temperatures lower than those accepted in surgical practice were used. *Bunker* and *Goldstein* [1] observed in man subjected to hypothermia a prolonged clotting time, although in their experience the concentration of the specific factors had remained practically unmodified during hypothermia (29.1° to 31° C), before the beginning of surgery and before the transfusion of blood. These authors reported 10 cases, 8 of which had undergone neurosurgical operations. The diagnoses were cerebral aneurysm (4 patients), meningioma (3 patients), cerebellar hemangioblastoma (1 patient). They carried out an analytical study on the main coagulation factors by measuring prothrombin activity, prothrombin consumption, factor V, factor VII, fibrinogen content, clotting time and platelet count.

The primary purpose of our researches was to estimate the effect of moderate hypothermia on coagulation and, secondarily, to determine coagulation changes during endocranial surgery and in the first postoperative days.

Changes in the specific factors of hemostasis will be studied later. At the present time, studies have been undertaken to evaluate coagulability from a general standpoint and to determine contemporaneously the prothrombin activity, which is the result of a complex balance of many specific factors.

Methods

The following laboratory studies were carried out:

Percent *prothrombin activity*, determined by the Quick method. It includes the action of prothrombin, of accelerating, converting and antagonizing factors. The normal value of prothrombin activity ranges between 70 and 105%.

Dextran sulfate tolerance test: This corresponds to the *in vitro* heparin tolerance test. Heparin solutions, due to their unstable activity and difficult preservation, were here replaced by dextran sulfate solution which show better stability and easier manipulation. General information on the hemocoagulatory balance is obtained by this test which is highly valuable because of its sensitivity both in hypocoagulability and hypercoagulability conditions. Practically, the clotting time is sensitized by addition of scalar amounts of dextran which interact in the complex of positive factors having antagonistic effect on coagulation.

Tests corresponding to 5, 10 and 15 minutes for 0.02, 0.04 and 0.05 dextran sulfate solutions respectively were regarded as normocoagulants; a shortening to 2 to 3 minutes at least was an indication of hypercoagulability, whereas a prolongation of 2 to 3 minutes at least was an indication of hypocoagulability.

4 *

Blood samples were withdrawn from the radial artery or from the median cubital vein under basal conditions, that is at the time of admission to hospital, and were taken again after induction of anesthesia, during hypothermia (esophageal temperature between 28° and 33°), intra- and post-operatively and in the following days.

Samples were obtained without a strict uniformity of time and temperature because of the variable individual conditions (more or less rapid fall of body temperature, more or less prolonged surgery).

The choice of the two above-mentioned tests has been suggested and conditioned by the imperative necessity of repeated determinations at short intervals.

Results

A great difficulty we met in our studies was the inability to obtain the lowest temperatures prior to surgery, blood transfusion or fluids infusion, conditions which surely influence blood co-agulation.

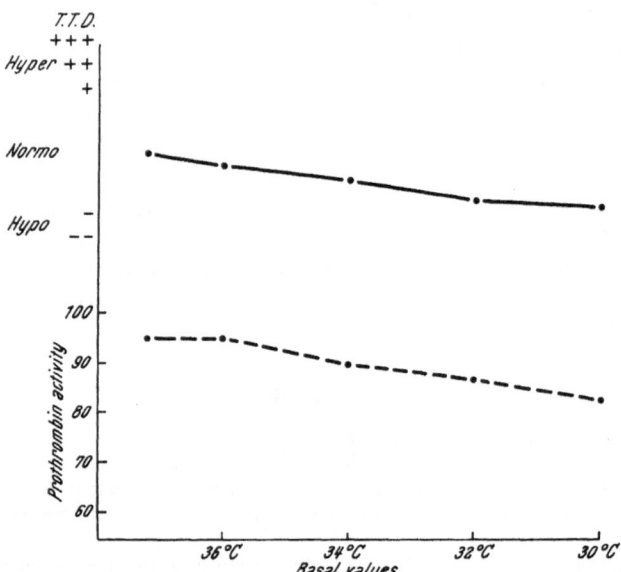

Fig. 1. Behaviour of the tolerance test and prothrombin activity during moderate hypothermia, before the intradural stage of the operation and before blood transfusions (7 cases)

Anaesthesia can also affect blood coagulation especially through influence on the vegetative nervous system. In 7 out of 25 control patients (20 had aneurysms) these influences could be nevertheless reduced to a minimum. Thus, controls carried out during gradual temperature falls revealed a progressive and constant (although not marked) prolongation of the dextran tolerance test values in association with a slight prothrombin hypoactivity. This finding was found in 6 of the 7 cases (Figs. 1 and 2). In most patients, controls performed just after the beginning of blood transfusion and surgery (especially in the intradural stage) showed a rapid modification of the dextran tolerance test, with a shift towards

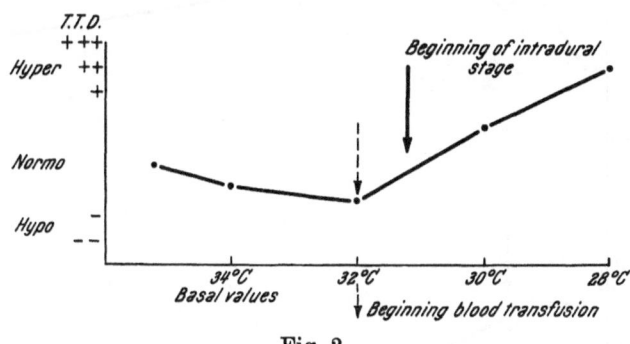

Fig. 2

values markedly shorter than basal levels. This appears to be in contrast with the prothrombin activity which showed, conversely, a further progressive drop.

In the remaining 18 cases intra- and post-operative controls failed to demonstrate an unequivocal behaviour of the dextran tolerance test. Indeed, on account of the effects of surgical procedures in general and of tissue manipulation in endocranial surgery, a marked shift towards hypercoagulability had to be expected. As a matter of fact, this was observed to a significant extent in a high percentage of the cases under observation (see Figs. 3 and 4). In other cases, however, there was no evidence

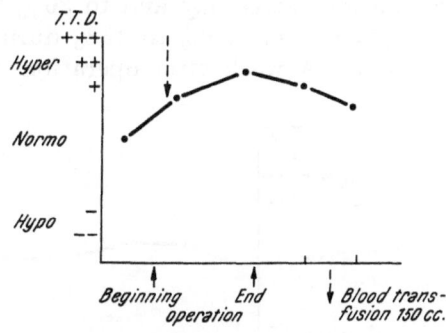

Fig. 3. Case 2 G.I. (anterior communicating artery aneurysm)

of significant changes (Fig. 5) and in two cases even hypocoagulability was demonstrated (Fig. 6) in spite of a reasonably moderate depression in prothrombin activity (Fig. 7).

The behaviour of prothrombin activity showed greater uniformity and was shown to undergo significant and lasting depression in a relevant number of patients. For example, in case No. 7 (Fig. 8) prothrombin activity dropped from 70% to 43% on the

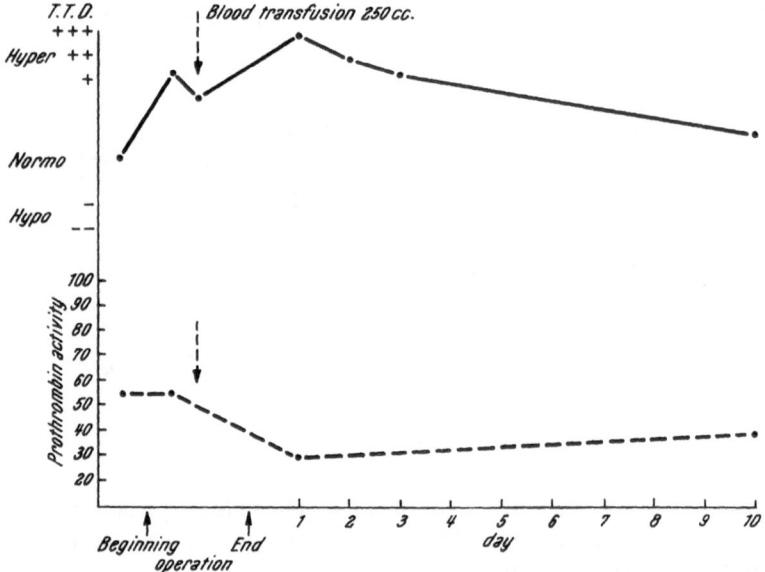

Fig. 4. Case 3 B.L. (anterior communicating artery aneurysm and left pre-central a.v. malformation)

first postoperative day and to 30% two days later. In case No. 9 it dropped from 100% to 45% during surgery and to 30% three days later. A week after operation it was still 40% (Fig. 9).

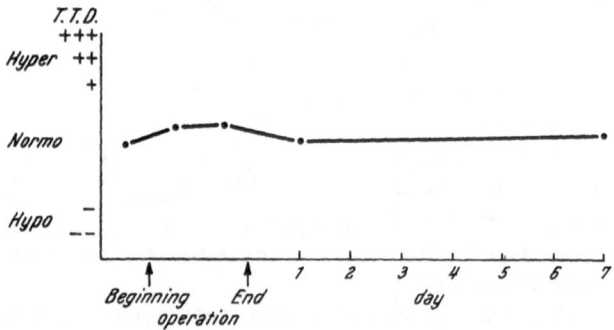

Fig. 5. Case 8 B.P. (olfactory groove meningioma)

Controls were carried out by the same procedure on a number of patients undergoing endocranial surgery at normal temperature.

Even in these cases, as already observed by many authors [7] [10] [11], and in cardiosurgical operations, as shown by investigators from our school (*Vergani, Panizzari* and *Sideri*) [9] evidence was obtained of the intra-operative appearance of total hypercoagulability and hypo-prothrombinemia which lasted for several days.

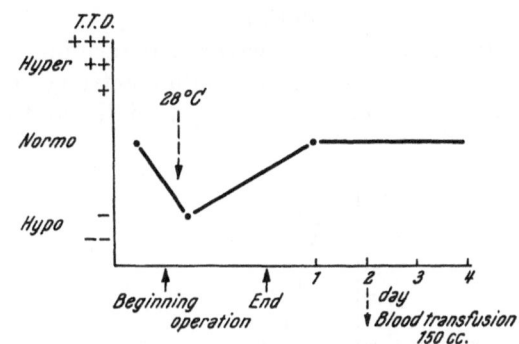

Fig. 6. Case 10 R.D. (aneurysm of the bifurcation anterior-middle cerebral arteries)

Conclusions

The observations described in this paper lead to the suggestion or confirmation of two main points: 1) a negative effect of body hypothermia on blood coagulation from a general standpoint; 2) a hypercoagulant effect of surgery (in this case of endocranial surgery).

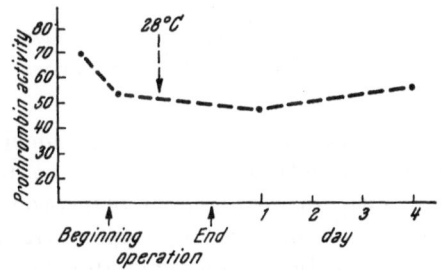

Fig. 7. Case 10 R.D.

Owing to the steadiness and uniformity of data, the first finding is no doubt significant, in spite of the small number of cases and of the fact that observations were confined to times not subjected to influences by the true initial surgery and blood transfusion.

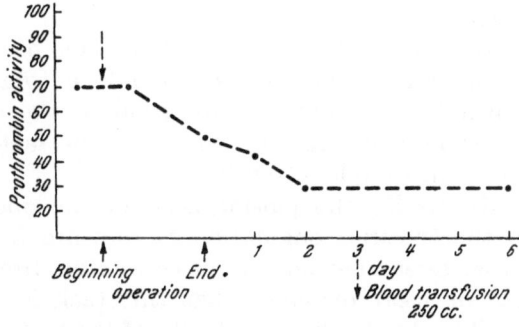

Fig. 8. Case 7 Z.G.B. (communicating artery aneurysm)

The early intra- and post-operative hypercoagulability was found to be less constant. Since hypercoagulability is a usual

consequence of surgical procedures in general, this value, lower
than that induced by any other operative procedure, may be
looked upon as the result of the depressant effect of hypothermia
upon blood coagulation.

In some cases, however, a determinant role was surely exerted
by the depressed prothrombin activity which was observed in a
large proportion of cases (especially at the beginning of the true

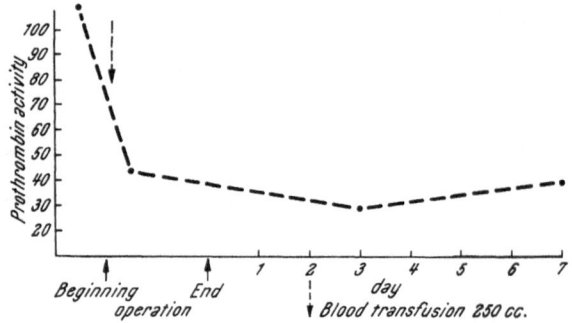

Fig. 9. Case 9 C.M. (communicating artery aneurysm)

surgical phase) and attained even remarkable values. Post-operative
prothrombin activity was shown to be rather singular in comparison with any other operative procedure. As a matter of fact,
hypoprothrombinemia develops rather frequently during any
surgical operation, but generally lessens and disappears in the
early post-operative phase. In a certain number of our patients
it persisted for a long period of time, being occasionally even
accentuated.

In case No. 7 (Fig. 8) the depression of the level of prothrombin
factors was so marked as to induce total hypocoagulability, as
shown by the marked alteration of the dextran tolerance test:
this showed changes in thrombophilic factors throughout surgery
and immediately after it.

To clarify the pathogenesis of the observed changes, studies
on the specific coagulation factors are first of all required. But
earlier researches both by investigators from our and other groups
provide clear evidence that this task is very hard or even impossible, due to the complexity of the factors involved and the lack
of uniformity of behaviour in each individual patient. Suggestions
as to the causes of hypocoagulability during hypothermia are easier
to make, if only we keep in mind the relevant effect of temperature
decrease upon the various *in vitro* clotting tests. As to the observed

hypoprothrombinemia, the extent to which it occurs suggests a more careful and through investigation, now under way.

All the evidence obtained would seem to justify the different evolutional possibilities of the intra- and post-operative course in patients predisposed both to thrombotic processes and haemorrhagic complications. In addition, it strongly supports the importance of a careful and frequent estimation of blood coagulability in patients undergoing the above-mentioned surgical procedures.

Summary

The author studied the behaviour of blood coagulation by dextran sulfate tolerance test *in vitro* and the prothrombin activity in 25 patients during neurosurgical operation under moderate hypothermia.

In 7 cases, in which it was possible to have data of hypothermic patients, after induction of anaesthesia but prior to surgery, there was observed a moderate hypocoagulability (demonstrated by a slight prolongation of the dextran sulfate tolerance test values in association, in 6 of the 7 cases, with a slight prothrombin hypoactivity).

In the remaining 18 cases, intra- and post-operative data generally evidenced a depression in prothrombin activity but failed to demonstrate an unequivocal behaviour of blood coagulation, as a whole.

Zusammenfassung

Die Autoren untersuchten das Verhalten der Blutgerinnung mit Hilfe des Dextran-sulfat-Toleranz-Tests in vitro und die Prothrombin-Aktivität bei 25 Patienten während neurochirurgischer Eingriffe in mäßiger Hypothermie.

Bei 7 Fällen, bei denen Werte hypothermierter Patienten zwar nach Einleitung der Narkose, aber vor Beginn der Operation zu erhalten waren, wurde eine mäßige Hypokoagulabilität festgestellt, gekennzeichnet durch eine geringe Verlängerung des Dextran-sulfat-Toleranz-Test-Wertes bei 6 von 7 Fällen, verbunden mit einer geringen Prothrombin-Hypoaktivität.

Bei den übrigen 18 Fällen ergaben die Werte während und nach der Operation zwar allgemein eine Minderung der Prothrombin-Aktivität, ließen aber insgesamt kein gleichförmiges Verhalten der Blutgerinnung erkennen.

Résumé

On a examiné les modifications de l'émocoagulation dans 25 sujets au cours des interventations neurochirurgicales en hypotermie modérée, au moyen du text de tolèrance au sulfate de dextrane et de l'activité prothrombinique.

On a observé, dans 7 patients, déjà soumis à l'anesthesie et au réfroidissement, mais pas encore à l'intervention, ipocoagulabilité modeste, et abaissement moderé de l'activité prothrombinique.

Dans les autres 18 cas, au cours de contrôles intra et post operatoires, on a observé généralement abaissement de l'activité prothrombinique, mais l'Auteur n'a pas décelé des modifications univoques de la coagulation globale du sang.

Riassunto

Sono state studiate le modificazioni della emocoagulabilità in 25 soggetti sottoposti ad intervento neurochirurgico in ipotermia moderata, mediante il test di tolleranza al solfato-destrano "in vitro" e l'attività protrombinica. In 7 pazienti anestetizzati e resi ipotermici sono state osservate modesta ipocoagulabilità e lieve abbassamento dell'attività protrombinica.

Negli altri 18 casi nei quali non è stato possibile effettuare prelievi prima dell'intervento, e stato possibile osservare nel corso dell'intervento stesso ed anche nei giorni seguenti abbassamento dell'attività protrombinica, ma non sono state notate modificazioni univoche della emocoagulabilità globale.

Resumen

Se han observado las modificaciones de la hemocoagulación en 25 sujetos en el curso de intervenciones neuroquirúrgicas bajo hipotermia moderada por medio de un test de tolerancia al sulfato de dextrano y de la actividad pro-trombínica.

Se ha visto en 7 enfermos, sometidos a la anestesia y al enfriamiento pero no todavía a la intervención, hipocoagulación moderada y un descenso moderado de la actividad protrombínica.

En los otros 18 casos, en los cuales no fué posible efectuar observaciones preoperatorias, pudimos observar en el curso de la intervención y en los dias siguientes un descenso de la actividad protrombínica, pero no se obser-varon modificaciones unívocas de la hemocoagulación global.

References

1) *Bunker, J. P.*, and *R. Goldstein.* (With Technical Assistance of *Amelia Yanakis.*) Coagulation during Hypothermia in man. Proceedings Soc. Exp. Biol. Med. *97* (1958), 199. — 2) *Fowler, N. O.:* Study of certain aspects of blood coagulation in postoperative state, in congestive heart failure and in thrombophlebitis. J. Clin. Invest. *3* (1951), 168. — 3) *Hagedorn, A. B.*, and *N. W. Barker:* Coagulation time of blood heparinized in vitro; correlation of results with those of heparin tolerance test. J. Lab. Clin. Med. *32* (1947), 1087. — 4) *Marmont, A.*, and *A. Palmieri:* Gli stati trombofilici. Diagnostica funzionale e concetti patogenetici. Medicina *1* (1951), 651. — 5) *Montini, T.*, *G. Paoletti* e *F. Piccinini:* Atti del XV° Symposium Internazionale sull'ipo-termia. Belgrado, 27 settembre — 5 ottobre 1937. — 6) *Paoletti, G.*, *T. Mon-tini* e *F. Piccinini:* Ultimi contributi allo studio della emocoagulabilità nella ipotermia sperimentale. Sperimentale *108/6* (1958), 531—538. — 7) *Scara-belli, L.*, e *G. Guagliano:* Applicazione del test all'urea per lo studio della coagulazione ematica nel periodo postoperatorio e durante il trattamento delle tromboflebiti. Atti Soc. Lomb. Sci. Med. Biol. *3* (1957), 439. — 8) *Silver-man, S. B.:* A modification of Waugh-Ruddick test for increased coagula-bility of the blood and its application to the study of postoperative case. Blood *3* (1948), 147. — 9) *Vergani, G.*, *G. P. Panizzari* e *G. C. Sideri:* Modifi-cazioni della coagulabilità ematica indotte dagli interventi chirurgici sul torace. Min. Med. *53*, n° 12 (1962), 386, 391. — 10) *Warren, R.*, *M. O. Admur,*

J. S. Belko, and *D. V. Baker, jr.*: Postoperative alterations in coagulation mechanism of blood: observations on circulating thromboplastin. Arch. Surg. *61* (1950), 419. — 11) *Warren, R.*, and *J. S. Belko*: Deficiency of plasma prothrombin conversion accelerators in postoperative state with description of simple method of assay. Blood *6* (1951), 544.

Clinica Medica — Università degli Studi — Milano (Italy)

Electrocardiographic Changes During Moderate Hypothermia and Intracranial Operations

By

G. Fiorelli

With 9 Figures

Introduction

The cardiovascular changes caused by surgical hypothermia are well known (*Bigelow* et al., 1950 [1]; *Hicks* et al., 1956 [2]; *Cordone* e *Parentela*, 1957 [3]; *Bigelow*, 1958 [4], *Sellick*, 1963 [5]; *Lougheed*, 1961 [6]).

As far as the electrocardiographic changes observed during moderate hypothermia for neuro-surgery, *Gunton* et al., 1956 [7], and *Smith*, 1956 [8], reported reduction of the cardiac rate, increase of the time of atrioventricular conduction and of the electrical systole. The ST segment was depressed or elevated and a progressive reduction and inversion of the T waves was also observed. Only 30% of the cases in *Gunton*'s series retained the sinus rhythm, while the other cases showed various disturbances of the rhythm (atrial tachycardia, wandering pacemaker, atrial flutter and fibrillation and, in two cases, ventricular fibrillation). Although they occurred very frequently during the hypothermia period, the atrial arrhythmias were not, in this series, responsible for serious hemodynamic modifications, and they were reversible. On the other hand *Somerville*, 1960 [9], in 150 patients undergoing cardiac surgery, observed during moderate hypothermia, the temporary return of sinus rhythm and the numerical reduction of the premature beats in cases of atrial fibrillation and of atrioventricular block.

The purpose of the present paper is to examine the electrocardiographic behaviour during moderate hypothermia in a non-homogeneous group of patients, without or with heart diseases, subjected to neurosurgical hypothermia.

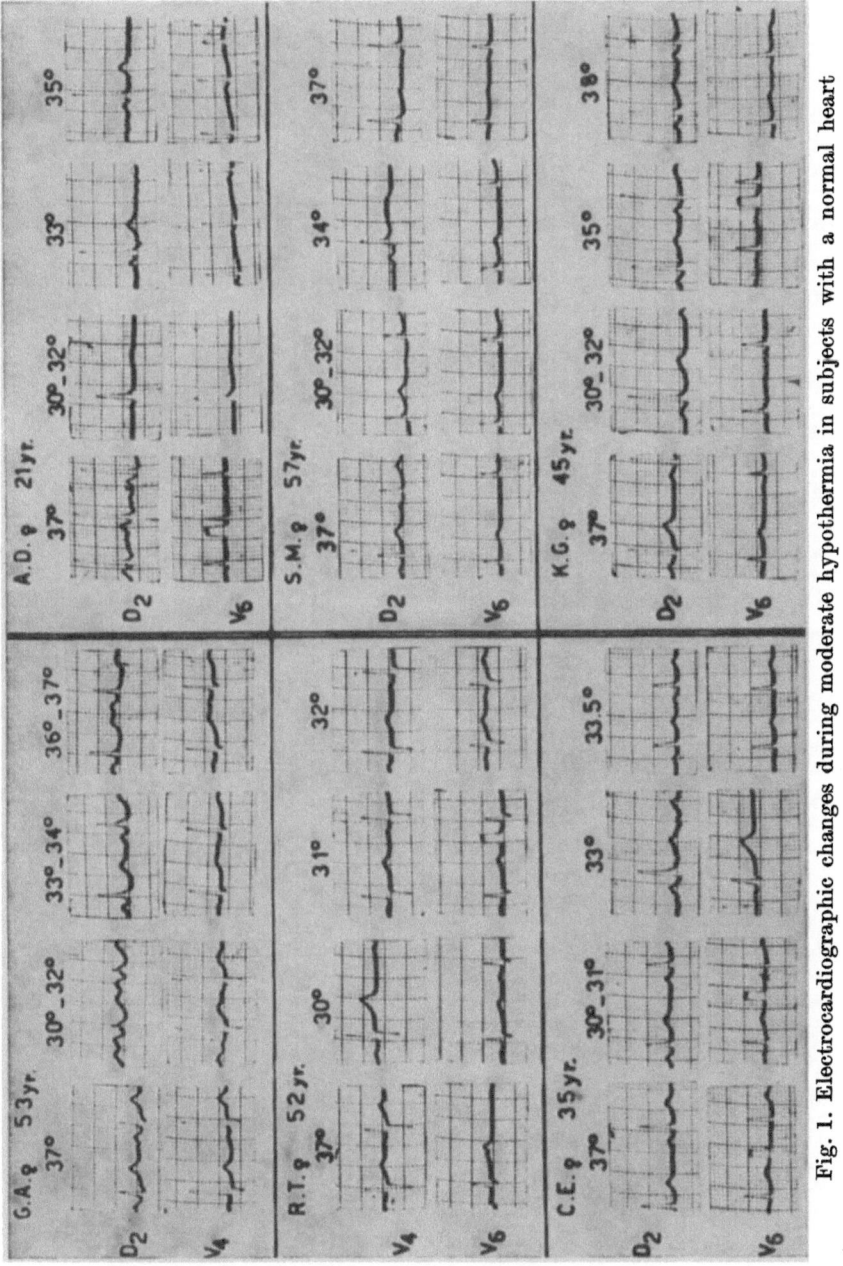

Fig. 1. Electrocardiographic changes during moderate hypothermia in subjects with a normal heart

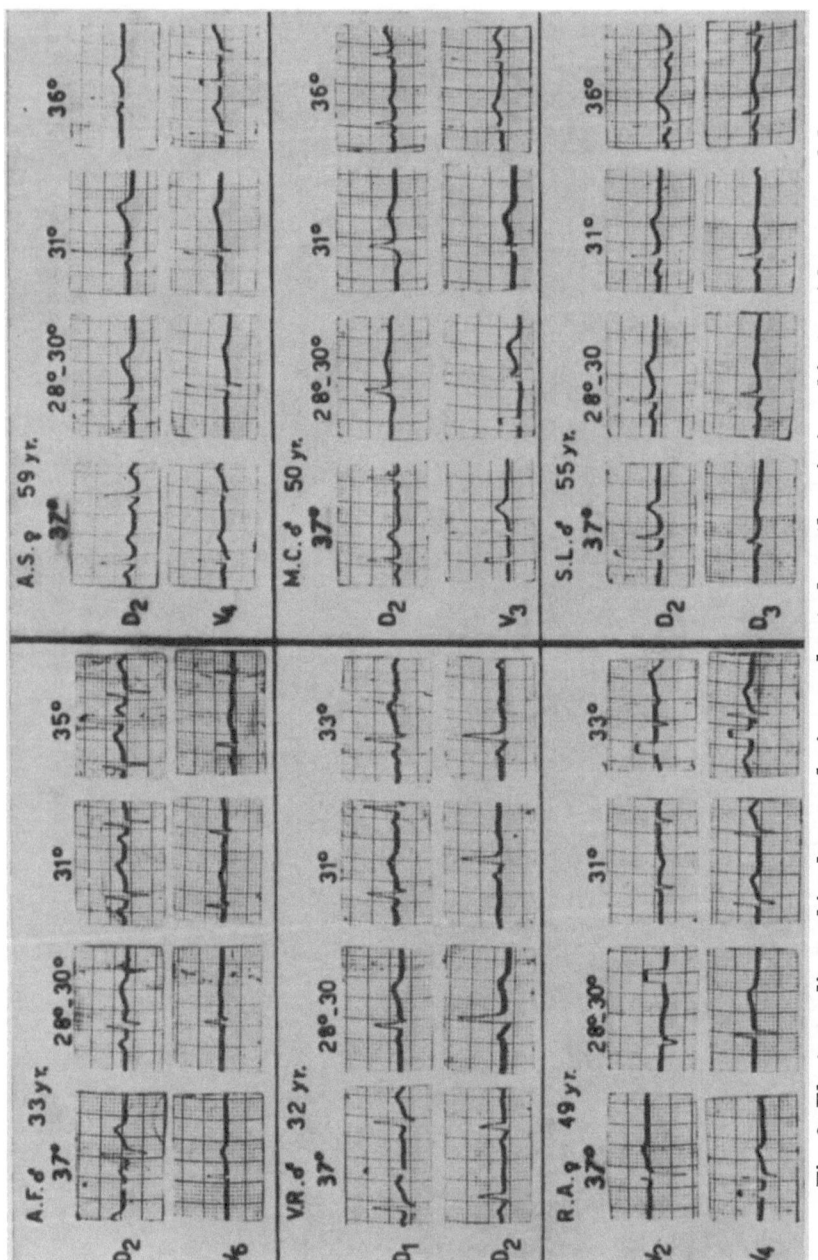

Fig. 2. Electrocardiographic changes during moderate hypothermia in subjects with a normal heart

Own Material

In this report 45 patients, ranging from 15 to 64 years of age, were studied. Heart diseases were present in 20 cases.

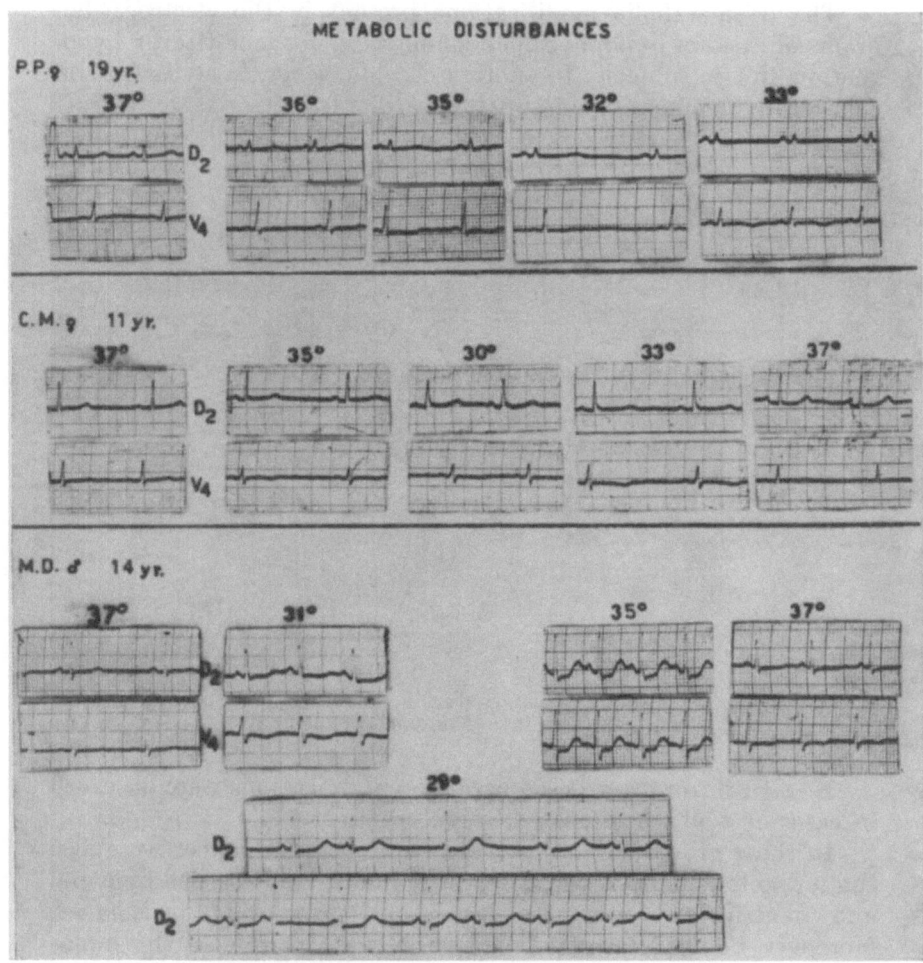

Fig. 3. Electrocardiographic changes during moderate hypothermia in cases of hypophysial adenoma: Metabolic disturbances

All the patients underwent electrocardiographic control before surgery, during the various stages of hypothermia and after return to normal temperature.

Results

Figs. 1 and 2 show the electrocardiographic changes revealed during hypothermia in normal subjects: reduction of the cardiac rate, increase of the PQ and QT, elevation of the ST segment and reduction of the T wave.

The dysmetabolic modifications present in the electrocardiograms of cases of hypophysial adenoma were not modified by hypothermia in two subjects. In another case, however, tachycardia and signs of involvement of the sub-endocardial layers, appeared during the heating stage (Fig. 3).

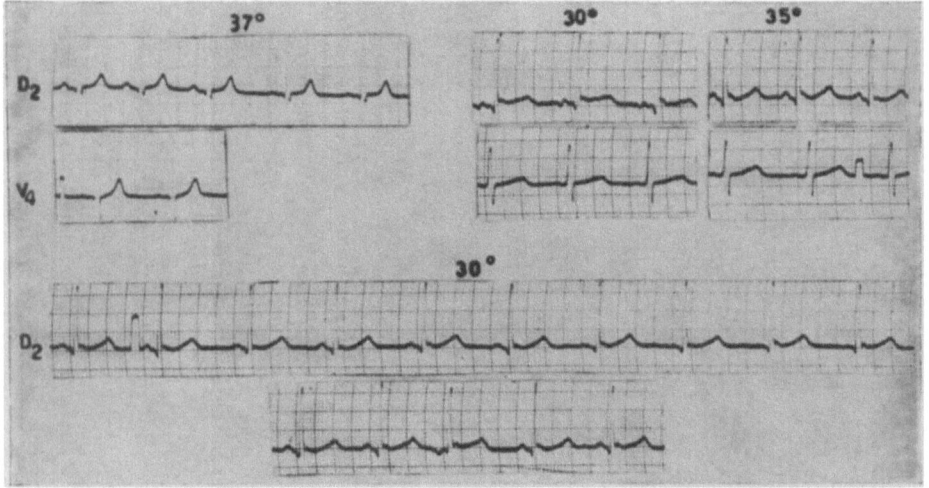

Fig. 4. Electrocardiographic changes during moderate hypothermia in cases with arrhythmias: Wandering pacemaker

No significant electrocardiographic modifications were observed in cases of well compensated valvulopathy.

In these groups of subjects the rhythm disturbances were also slight and low in incidence. They were mainly represented by atrial and ventricular premature beats and wandering pacemaker. Moreover, no changes were observed in cases in which arrhythmias were present before the hypothermia (Fig. 4 and Fig. 5).

The electrocardiographic modifications during hypothermia in cases with myocardial sclerosis and coronary insufficiency appear more interesting.

The incidence of arrhythmias was undoubtedly higher. The most frequent arrhythmias were atrial and ventricular premature beats and atrial fibrillation. Cases of ventricular fibrillation were never seen (Fig. 6 and Fig. 7). As regards the disturbances of conduction, the PQ and QRS times were increased. The changes of the repolarization waves, sometimes seen during the heating stage were all

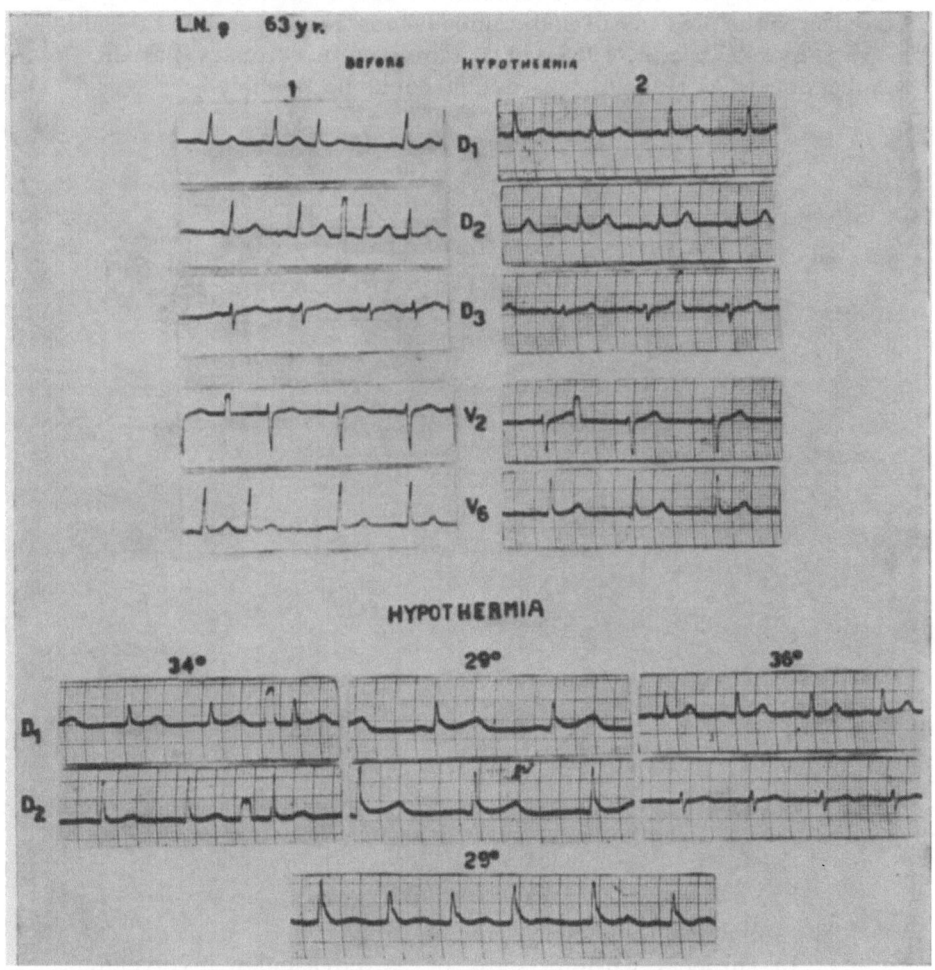

Fig. 5. Electrocardiographic changes during moderate hypothermia in cases with arrhythmias: Paroxysmal atrial fibrillation

reversible, regressing in the immediate post-operative period or during the following days (Fig. 8 and Fig. 9).

Compared with other series reported in the literature, our results have revealed an extremely low incidence and severity of alterations in rhythm, particularly in the cooling stage. This is probably refer-

able to the particular care with which the ventilatory process is
followed during this stage. The repolarization modifications observed
during the heating stage must probably be ascribed to the metabolic
and electrolytic variations (*Kaminer* and *Bernstein*, 1957 [10]), as
well as to the presence of non-homogeneous transmyocardial thermic
gradients (*Gillmann*, 1958 [11]). However in coronary patients a
subendocardial transitory ischemia could be possible.

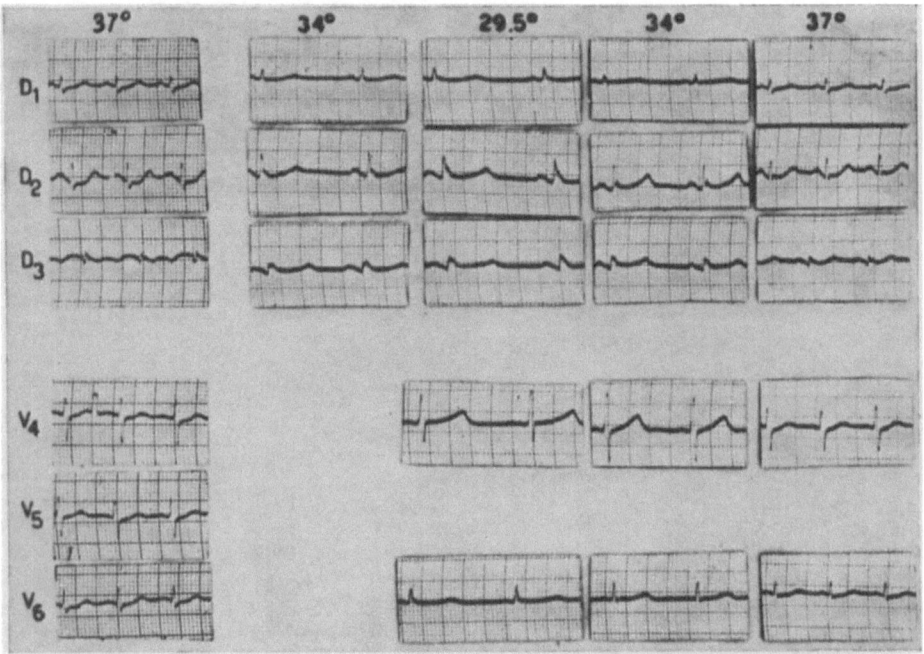

Fig. 6. Electrocardiographic changes during moderate hypothermia in a subject with coronary atherosclerosis

Conclusions

The following conclusions can be drawn:

1) In subjects without signs of cardiovascular involvement,
the electrocardiographic modifications produced during hypothermia
observed in our series of 45 cases are similar to the findings already
reported in the literature: bradycardia, increase of the atrioventricular conduction time, lengthening of the electrical systole and modification of the ST segment, generally upwards. Wandering pacemaker, atrial and ventricular premature beats rarely appeared.

2) In the group with heart diseases the arrhythmias appeared
more frequently in subjects with symptoms of coronary insufficiency

particularly during the terminal stage of hypothermia, and were mainly represented by atrial and ventricular premature beats and by atrial fibrillation (no cases of ventricular fibrillation were observed). Finally modifications of the repolarization wave (flattening or inversion of the T wave) were observed in some cases, particularly during the heating stage, and these might be ascribed to ischemic disturbances or involvement of the sub-endocardiac layers, although

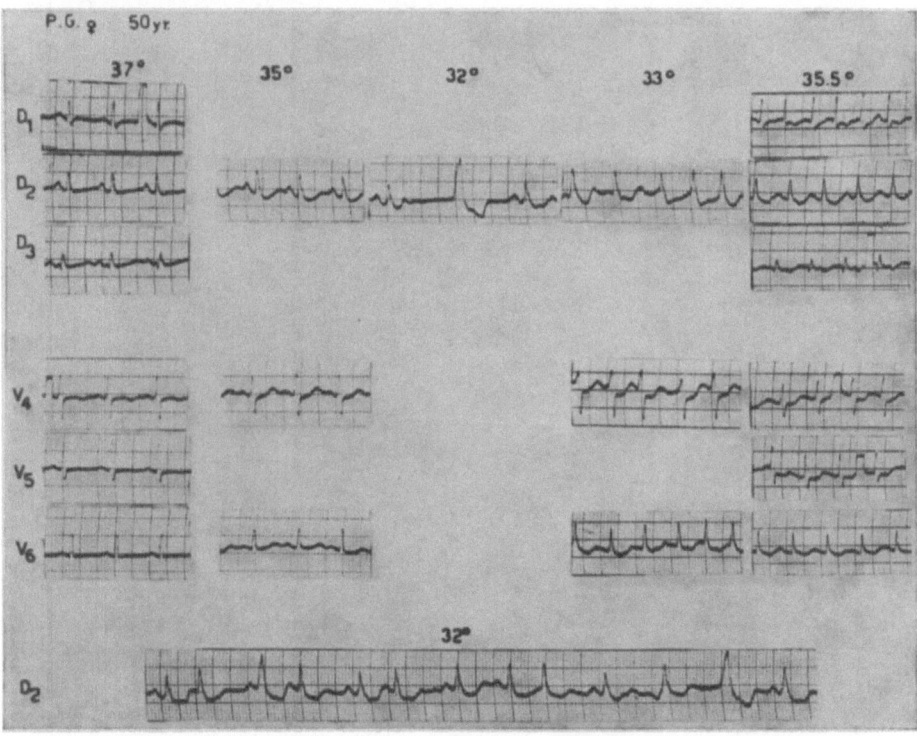

Fig. 7. Electrocardiographic changes during moderate hypothermia in a subject with coronary insufficiency

always of reversible nature. We should emphasize that these findings tend to regress in the immediate post-operative period, lasting a few days at the most.

Summary

The electrocardiographic changes during moderate hypothermia in neurosurgical patients were studied. The appearance of some arrhythmias during hypothermia was more frequent in subjects with heart disease than in cases with a normal heart. In subjects

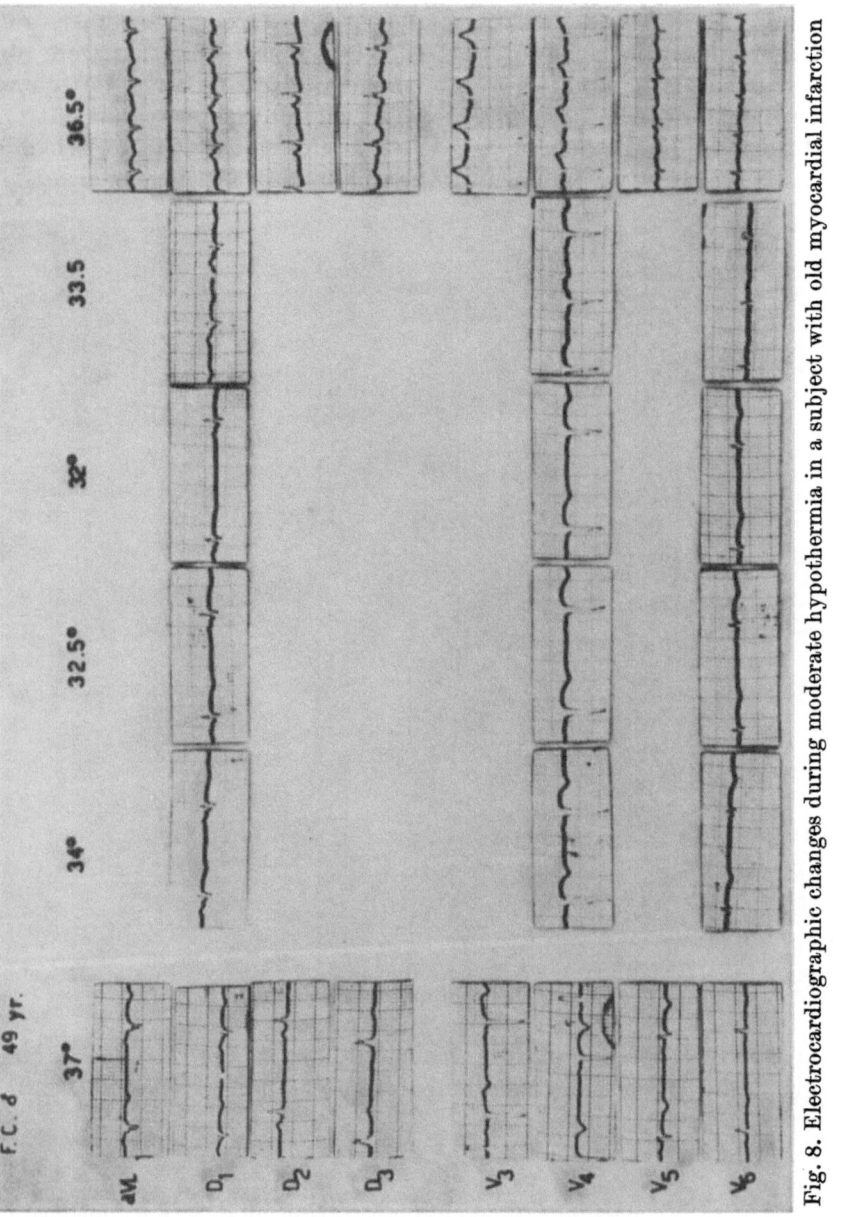

Fig. 8. Electrocardiographic changes during moderate hypothermia in a subject with old myocardial infarction

with coronary heart disease modifications of the repolarization waves were observed in some cases. These changes might be ascribed

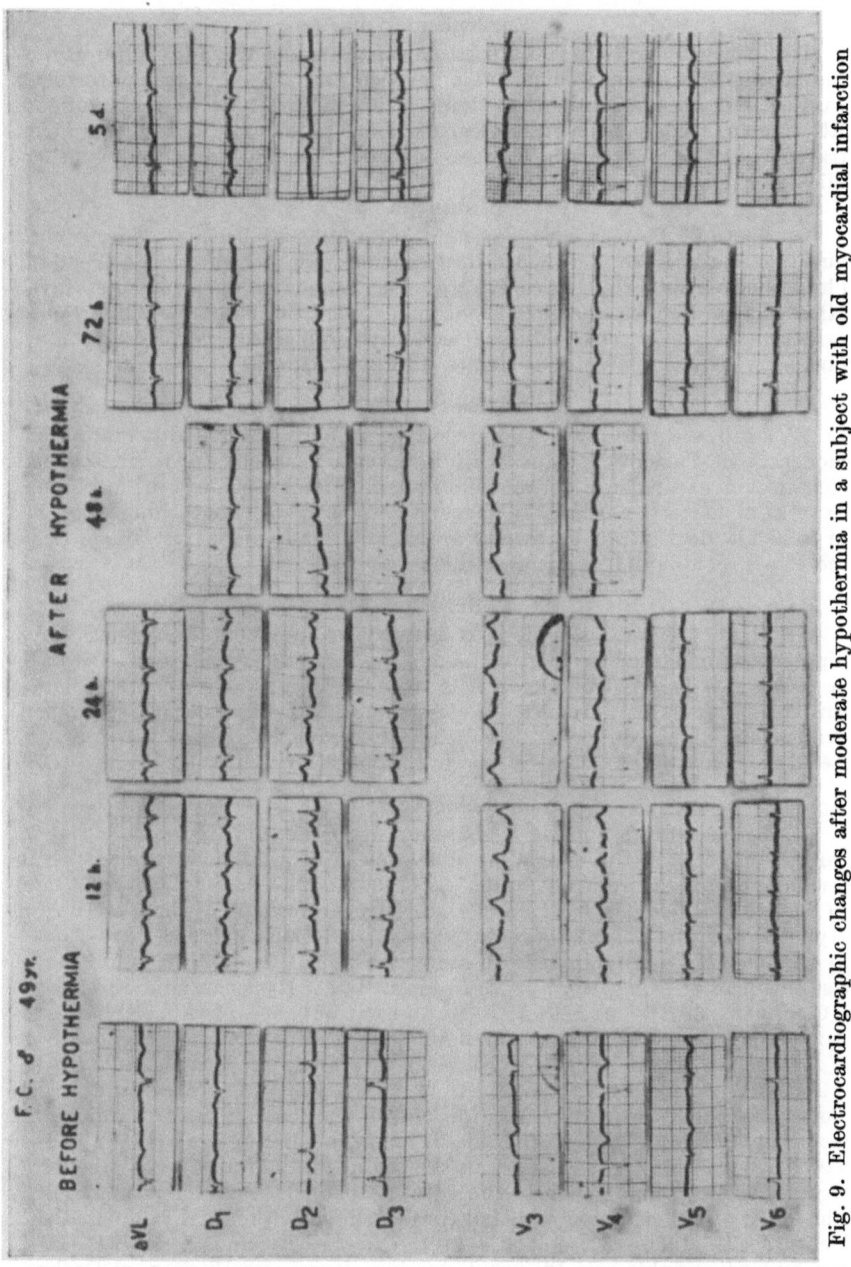

Fig. 9. Electrocardiographic changes after moderate hypothermia in a subject with old myocardial infarction

to ischemic disturbances or involvement of the sub-endocardial layers, although always of reversible nature.

Zusammenfassung

Der Autor untersucht das Elektrokardiogramm während leichter Hypothermie bei Patienten, welche einem neurochirurgischen Eingriff unterzogen wurden. Herzkranke Patienten zeigten während der Hypothermie häufigere Rhythmusstörungen als Normalpersonen. Bei Kranken mit Coronarstörungen traten reversible ischemische Zeichen auf, vor allem am Ende der Hypothermie.

Résumé

On a étudié l'électrocardiogramme durant l'hypothermie modérée chez quelques malades soumis à des interventions neurochirurgicales. Pendant l'hypothermie les arhythmies étaient plus fréquentes chez les sujets avec affections cardiaques que chez les normaux. Chez les sujets coronaires on a évidencié des signes d'ischémie sous-endocardiaque avec caractère réversible, plus souvent dans les phases finales de l'hypothermie.

Riassunto

E' stato eseguito uno studio elettrocardiografico durante l'ipotermia moderata in Pazienti sottoposti ad interventi neurochirurgici. In soggetti con affezioni cardiache le aritmie sono state più numerose, durante l'ipotermia, rispetto ai soggetti normali. In soggetti coronaropatici sono comparsi segni di ischemia degli strati sottoendocardici, più spesso nella fase finale della ipotermia, con carattere di reversibilità.

Resumen

En algunos enfermos sometidos a intervenciones neuroquirúrgicas bajo hipotermia moderada se han estudiado los electrocardiogramas. Durante la hipotermia las arritmias eran más frecuentes en aquellos con afecciones cardiacas que en los normales. En sujetos con afecciones coronarias se han evidenciado dignos de isquemia subendocárdica de caracter reversible, más frecuentemente en las fases finales de la hipotermia.

References

1) *Bigelow, W. C.*, and *W. K. Lindsay:* Hypothermia. Its possible role in cardiac surgery; an investigation of factors governing survival in dogs at low body temperature. Ann. Surg. *132* (1950), 849—866. — 2) *Hicks, C. E.*, *M. C. McCord*, and *S. G. Blount, Jr.:* Electrocardiographic Changes During Hypothermia and Circulatory Occlusion. Circulation *13* (1956), 21—28. — 3) *Cordone, M.*, e *A. Parentela:* L'ipotermia — E.M.E.S., Edizioni mediche e scientifiche — Roma, 1957. — 4) *Bigelow, W. C.:* Hypothermia. Surgery *43* (1958), 683—687. — 5) *Sellick, B. A.:* Recent advances in Anaesthesia and Analgesia, p. 111. London: C. Langton Hewer Ed. 1963. — 6) *Lougheed, W. M.:* The Central Nervous System in Hypothermia. Brit. Med. Bull. *17* (1961), 61—65. — 7) *Gunton, R., J. W. Scott, W. M. Lougheed*, and *E. H. Botterell:* Changes in cardiac rhythm and in the form of electrocardiogram resulting from induced hypothermia in man. Am. Heart J. *52* (1956), 419—429. — 8) *Smith, D. E.:* Changes in the electrocardiogram during preoperative hypothermia in man. Aust. Ann. Med. *5* (1956), 62—67. — *Somerville, W.:* The effect of hypothermia on atrial fibrillation and other arrhythmias. Brit. Heart J. *22* (1960), 515—521. — 10) *Kaminer, B.*, and *E. R. Bernstein:* Electrocardiographic and Plasma Potassium Responses Elicited on Cooling the Chest Wall of Man. Circulation *15* (1957), 559—567. — 11) *Gillmann, H. I.:* Vektorielle Untersuchungen über die durch künstliche Hypothermie ausgelösten EKG-Veränderungen. Cardiologia *33* (1958), 21—31.

Servizio di Anestesia e Rianimazione — Clinica Neurochirurgica — Università degli Studi — Milano (Italy)

Methods of Moderate Hypothermia in Neuroanaesthesia. Clinical Observations on Physiological and Metabolic Changes

By

M. Bozza Marrubini, A. Visca, L. Tretola, and G. Signoroni

With 19 Figures

Introduction

Moderate hypothermia has been used for many years and by many authors for neurosurgical operations.

At first the main points of interest discussed were the technical problems, both anaesthesiological and physical, the safety and limits of the new technique, as well as its effects on brain volume, function, metabolism and circulation.

After nearly a decade of clinical use a great mass of data has been published and, with few exceptions, general agreement has been reached on many points; general reviews have been published in which the problems of heat transfer during surface cooling and during extracorporeal cooling, those of temperature monitoring and of thermoregulation block are clearly discussed and settled (see *Verbiest*, 1956; *Virtue*, 1955; *Dundee* and *King*, 1959; *Little*, 1959; *Cooper* and *Ross*, 1960; *Boba*, 1960).

With the increase of clinical experience the general interest has shifted to other complex problems, such as the choice of the best cooling technique among the great number of methods described, the prediction of the cooling rate and temperature after drop and the choice of anaesthetic agents and supplementary drugs.

Moreover, up to date no agreement has been reached whether it is safer and preferable to associate hypothermia with induced hypotension or with temporary arrest of cerebral circulation; in addition there is no agreement on the characteristics and on the evaluation of the severity of respiratory, metabolic and cardiovascular manifestations subsequent to the induction of moderate hypothermia, nor on the best way to prevent and control these changes.

Opinions differ widely also about the safe period of cerebral circulatory occlusion at the temperatures of moderate hypothermia: clinical data seem to indicate that cerebral ischemia in the hypothermic anaesthetized patient may be tolerated for longer periods of time than could be predicted from experimental data on the depression of cerebral metabolism in moderate hypothermia.

The aim of the present report is to describe the technical and anaesthesiological observations made during a six-years' experience with moderate hypothermia in neurosurgery, and to contribute to the discussion and solution of some of the above mentioned problems.

1. Technical Problems

Moderate hypothermia in neurosurgery is usually obtained by surface cooling. Other methods such as intragastric cooling (*Khalil*, 1957 and 1958; *Holt* et al., 1958; *Barnard*, 1956) or extra-corporeal veno-venous cooling (*Foltz* and *Frederickson*, 1960) have been described, but up to now their use has not known wide diffusion.

The *physical principles* of surface cooling can be briefly summarized as follows.

For heat exchanges, the temperature differential (Θ) between the body and the cooling system (blanket, mattress, ice-bags, water or air), the area of the exposed surface (S) and the heat transfer coefficient (K) must be taken into account.

The temperature differential can be varied at will, but for clinical use is usually kept in the range of $15-30°$ C.

The highest temperature differences between the patient's body and the cooling system occur when solid cooling materials (ice-bags, refrigerated blankets, ecc.) are employed.

The area of the body surface exposed to the cooling system is largest when a fluid is employed; when ice-bags, blankets or even rubber suits are used, only limited areas of the body surface and of the cooling surface adhere intimately, while the heat transmission of large portion of the body surface is impaired by a layer of still air with a very low heat transfer coefficient interposing between the cooling means and the body.

If the body is immersed in a fluid cooling medium, a much more continuous and intimate contact is obtained; but if the fluid is stagnant, or moving as a slow current with laminar flow, the heat exchange is very low owing to the low heat transfer coefficient of fluids in such conditions.

The heat transfer coefficient increases sharply if the fluid is kept moving turbulently (*Clutton-Brock*, 1959; *Mortimer*, 1957; *Vadot*, 1962).

The general formula for heat exchange is: —

$$Q = K.\ S.\ \Theta,$$

where Q is the heat flow and $K.$, $S.$ and Θ have been defined above.

This clearly shows that a higher temperature differential is necessary when the area of the cooling surface is relatively small, while, if S and K have high values, as happens when the patient is immersed in turbulently moving water or air, a rapid temperature fall may be obtained with a reduced temperature differential (*Bozza* and *Rossanda*, 1962; *Wyndham* et al., 1959; *Forrester*, 1958; *Clutton-Brock*, 1959; *Williams*, 1962).

The air heat transfer coefficient is lower than the water coefficient (*Vadot*, 1962); therefore the maintenance of a turbulent flow is more important in cooling methods using air chambers than in methods employing a cold bath.

The living body subjected to active cooling however does not behave simply as a physical body (*von Euler*, 1961; *Waters* and *Mapleson*, 1961). Heat conduction within the outer surface and the inner parts of the living organism is greatly influenced by the existence of blood circulation (*Delorme*, 1956; *Wissler*, 1961).

Dhruva et al. (1963) have shown that the temperature fall obtained by immersion in cold water is much faster in a living animal than in a dead one; if the circulation is temporarily arrested by cardioplegia, the cooling rate is reduced; when the heart activity and blood circulation are restored the internal temperature falls again at a faster rate.

The importance of the peripheral circulation has been stressed by many authors using surface cooling, and all agree that anaesthetic and supplementary drugs having a powerful vasodilating action are most suitable for hypothermic anaesthesia.

Neurosurgical operations for which moderate hypothermia is required leave most of the body surface free for heat exchanges, so that, with suitable apparatus, surface cooling and rewarming can at least in part be accomplished during surgical manipulation.

Since general body cooling (and eventually rewarming) is a relatively slow process, the time of additional anaesthesia can be shortened if the temperature fall can be exactly timed with the preliminary extracranial phases of the operation.

For these reasons many authors have described cooling techniques which do not interfere with surgery: ice-bags (*Hellings*, 1958; *Sedzimir* and *Dundee*, 1958), refrigerated blankets or mattresses (*Cohen* and *Hercus*, 1959) inflatable plastic tubs or swimming pools placed on the operating table (*Bayuk* and *Chen*, 1961; *Gardner*, *Wasmuth*, and *Hale*, 1956; *Hebert* and *Merzig*, 1958; *Holswade* and *Engle*, 1958), refrigerated rubber suits (*Oppeln-Bronikowsky*, 1962) even a special surgical table with a closed circuit cold air cabinet enclosing the patient up to the neck (Auto-Hypotherm of *Adams-Ray* and *Persson*, *Adams-Ray*, 1958).

Even if the classical method of immersion in cold water in an ordinary bath-tub is used, the operation can begin long before the body temperature has reached its lowest point; as this method has a very marked after drop, active cooling must be discontinued very early; as soon as the temperature has reached 33—32° C the patient is lifted from the bath and can be positioned on the operating table, so that surgery can proceed during the second part of the cooling process.

Few authors have paid attention to the actual lengthening of the total anaesthetic time due to the use of hypothermia. From the available data the additional anaesthetic time appears to be not less than one hour (*Cooper* and *Ross*, 1960) extending in many cases to two or even three hours. As neurosurgical operations for which hypothermia is employed are usually lengthy procedures (aneurysms, large angiomas or meningiomas, craniopharyngiomas, etc.) it may be necessary to maintain anaesthesia for nine — ten hours or even longer (*Millet* and *Viale-Millet*, 1962).

This fact must be borne in mind when an attempt to evaluate the different cooling and anaesthesiological techniques is made.

The control of the final temperature level is closely linked with the choice of the cooling technique.

All surface cooling methods give a faster temperature fall in the peripheral parts of the body (*Cooper* and *Ross*'s "shell") than in the intra-abdominal, intrathoracic and intracranial contents (the "core"). When cooling is stopped there is a redistribution of heat between the core and the shell which leads to a continuing drop in deep body temperature, named "after drop".

If not exactly controlled this phenomenon may lead to serious troubles, as the safety margin between surgical hypothermia (31—28° C) and the temperature level at which cardio-circulatory insufficiency is the rule (27—26° C) is very narrow (*Currie* et al.,

1962; *Lofstrom*, 1959; *Bigelow*, 1958; *Badeer*, 1962). As a matter of fact, most of the fatal or nearly-fatal cardiac accidents described by the authors who have first employed this technique in neuro-surgery were caused by an uncontrollable after drop in the patient's body temperature beyond the safety limit.

Some authors have tried to find general rules by which the after drop could be exactly predicted (*Hamilton*, 1960; *Boba*, 1960; *Forrester* and *Brown*, 1961) but, as complex calculations or tabu-lation of data are seldom feasible in the operating rooms, the most accepted procedure is to keep rewarming means at hand during the operation (heated blankets or mattresses, thermostatically con-trolled or not) so that the temperature fall can be quickly stopped and reversed if necessary (*Sellick*, 1957; *Adams* and *Wylie*, 1959; *Boba*, 1960; *Campkin* and *Inglis*, 1958).

These problems may explain why, besides the earlier techniques, employing ice-packs or a cold water tub, increasingly complex, cumbersome and expensive apparatuses have been devised.

As far as the *anaesthetic technique* is concerned it is generally agreed that, unless supplementary drugs such as muscle relaxants and/or phenothiazine are used, a fairly deep anaesthesia level is necessary in order to obtain a satisfactory block of thermoregula-tion reflexes and hence a regular temperature fall.

The importance of a complete block of thermoregulation has been stressed by all authors using hypothermic anaesthesia in man: if hypermetabolic and cardiovascular reactions and visible or invis-ible (*Froese*, 1958) shivering are allowed to occur, the temperature fall is greatly slowed (*Barila* and *Slocum*, 1955); moreover thermo-regulation reflexes are the cause of untoward cardiovascular alter-ations (*Hewer*, 1962; *Pool* and *Kessler*, 1958) and of severe acid-base regulation changes such as metabolic acidosis (*Fairley* et al., 1957).

Only *Mellinger* (1960) on the basis of an experimental study on small animals and *Waters* and *Mapleson* (1961) on man state that "oxygen consumption and heat production play a minor role in hypothermic anaesthesia and that the heat exchange on the body shell is the important factor".

This statement must be considered with great caution under clinical conditions: it must be remembered here that the main purpose of hypothermic anaesthesia is to obtain a reduction of oxygen consumption; if thermoregulation reflexes, with the resultant increased metabolic rate, are left active the true aim of hypothermia is lost, no matter if the increased heat production can be easily overcome by the more efficient cooling methods.

It must be stressed therefore that *all* thermoregulation reflexes must be blocked: both those which impair heat loss (vasoconstriction) and those which increase heat production (shivering and sympathetic activation).

The effects of the anaesthetic agents and of the supplementary drugs, commonly used for the induction of hypothermia, on the thermoregulation reflexes and on the cardiovascular system are illustrated in Fig. 1.

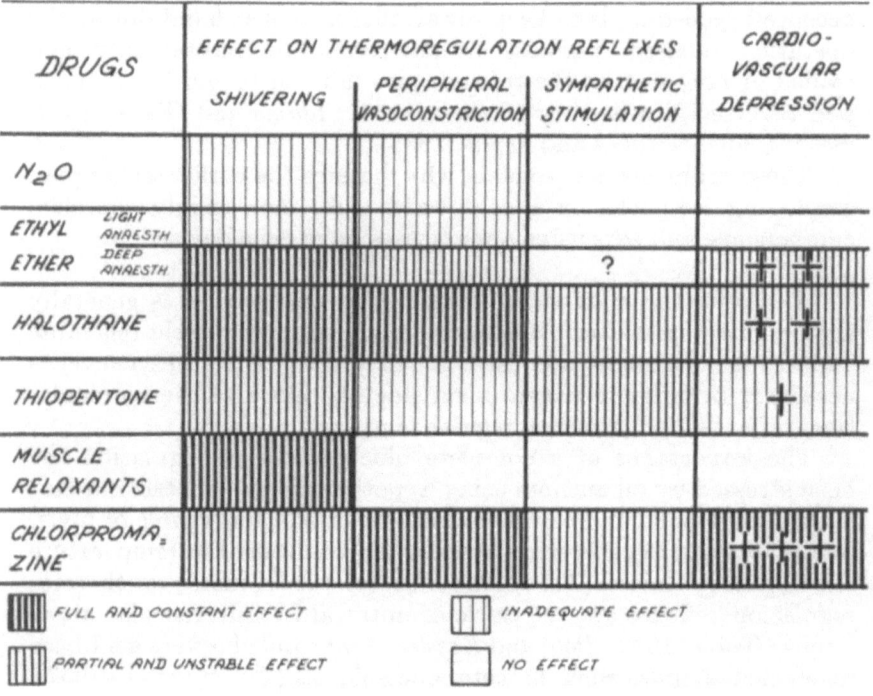

Fig. 1. Choice of drugs for the induction of hypothermia, with reference to their effects on thermoregulation reflexes and on the cardiovascular system.
+ Occasional cardiovascular depression
++ Moderate cardiovascular depression
+++ Severe cardiovascular depression

Nitrous oxide alone is inadequate to obtain a complete block; even its effect on shivering (*Sellick*, 1957; *Parkhouse*, 1957) has been recently denied (*Riabov*, 1962).

Deep ethyl ether anaesthesia gives a fairly complete block but cannot be used in neuroanaesthesia because of its untoward effects on brain volume and tension, on acid-base regulation (*Stevenson*, 1960) and on respiratory and circulatory balance.

"Light ether" as used in neuroanaesthesia (2—4% of vapour volume in inspired gases) does not affect vital functions or the intracranial operative field, but has an insufficient effect on vasoconstriction (*Waters* and *Mapleson*, 1961) while it may stimulate sympathetic activity; visible shivering is usually blocked, but invisible shivering and muscular rigidity are nearly always the rule when the internal temperature has dropped by 1 or 2° C.

Halothane approaches the ideal for hypothermic anaesthesia (*Borroni*, 1962; *Vandewater* et al., 1958; *Campkin* and *Inglis*, 1958; *Bayuk* and *Chen*, 1961) but its side effects on respiration and blood pressure must be carefully controlled (*Holmdahl* and *Payne*, 1960; *Dam*, 1960).

Vandewater et al. (1958) and *Bayuk* and *Chen* (1961) state that with halothane satisfactory anaesthesia for hypothermia can be obtained without any appreciable risk of cardiovascular and respiratory depression. *Borroni* and *Bozza Marrubini* (1962) claim better results when halothane is used with controlled respiration.

All authors however agree that with halothane an appreciable increase in the cooling rate can be obtained, probably through its peripheral vasodilating effect.

Dhruva et al. (1961) have shown that, with halothane anaesthesia, total circulatory occlusion may be prolonged beyond the accepted maximum times, both during normothermia and during hypothermia, without causing anoxic brain damage; the protective effect is obtained with fairly high concentrations and may be due to the reduction of total body oxygen consumption observed during halothane anaesthesia (*Krantz* et al., 1958; *Orton* and *Morris*, 1959).

If the observations of *Dhruva* et al. could be confirmed in man halothane would be the best agent available up to date for hypothermic anaesthesia.

Thiopentone is generally used for induction only, as most authors fear to use large doses of intravenous agents, whose detoxification and elimination are slowed in hypothermia (*Delorme*, 1956).

Only *Pool* and *Kessler* (1958) and *Purpura* et al. (1958) point out that thiopentone may be useful during hypothermia for the prevention and treatment of cardiac arrhythmias of reflex origin.

Chlorpromazine, because of its central effect on thermal regulation and its peripheral vasodilating action, is widely employed both as a premedicant and as a supplementary drug during hypothermic anaesthesia (*Dundee* et al., 1954; *Burrows* et al., 1956; *Millet* and *Viale-Millet*, 1962; *Jackson* et al., 1959; *Dundee*, 1954); its value is limited by its undesirable and unpredictable side effects on circulation (*Jackson* et al., 1959; *Rollason* and *Hough*, 1960).

Curarization, usually by d-tubocurarine, is used by some authors in order to block shivering without having recourse to deep general anaesthesia or to high doses of intravenous chlorpromazine.

Zaimis et al. (1958) and *Clutton-Brock* (1959) have pointed out that the action of competitive neuromuscular blocking drugs is reduced during hypothermia while excretion is delayed. This could lead to unexpected recurarization during rewarming. However, up to date no trouble of this type has been described.

The association of tubocurarine with halothane seems to be less dangerous than previously described (*Chatas* et al., 1963); in susceptible cases toxiferine may be a satisfactory substitute (*Foldes* et al., 1961).

2. Pathophysiological Problems

The general pattern of respiratory, acid-base and circulatory changes which follow moderate hypothermia has been described by *Rossanda* in the first chapter of this report.

Changes occurring in *acid-base regulation* during hypothermic anaesthesia have been the object of many experimental and clinical studies.

During hypothermia *cardiac arrhythmias* and *ventricular fibrill-ation* are closely related to *biochemical changes* (*Galindo* et al., 1962; *Beavers* and *Covino*, 1959); similarly during rewarming *metabolic acidosis* may lead to serious cardiovascular troubles and even to coma and irreversible shock (*Fairley* et al., 1957; *Bernard* et al., 1961; *Boeré*, 1962; *Bigelow*, 1959).

These problems are most important for cardiovascular surgery where the metabolic changes due to total circulatory arrest are added to those due to hypothermia. The picture may be further complicated by the effects of direct surgical manipulation of the heart and by changes due to extracorporeal artificial circulation with cardiopulmonary by-pass.

The results of experimental and clinical studies on hypothermia for this type of surgery are therefore scarcely indications for hypothermic anaesthesia in neurosurgery.

Total cerebral circulatory arrest has negligible effects on the general metabolic balance.

On the other hand most operations for which moderate hypothermia is indicated, require also the use of artifices in order to obtain an actual retraction of the brain as a whole; some of these artifices, as for instance the infusion of hypertonic urea or the maintenance of artificial hyperventilation, unavoidably upset metabolic or acid-base balance.

The main difficulty in the prevention and treatment of biochemical changes related to hypothermic anaesthesia is, as already pointed out by *Severinghaus* (1957), that it is impossible to define exactly the"normal" or optimal values for biochemical data during hypothermia.

The definition of the best acid-base conditions in patients under hypothermic anaesthesia has therefore given rise to many discussion.

Up to about 1960 most authors stated that as cardiac irregularities and post-hypothermic circulatory failure are related to the fall of blood pH due to hypothermia, an essential feature of the anaesthesiological management was the maintenance of a respiratory alkalosis obtained by *over-ventilation* (*Cooper* and *Ross*, 1960; *Virtue*, 1955; *Virtue* and *Wittenstein*, 1959; *Boeré*, 1956; *Barila* and *Slocum*, 1955). Only *Niazi* and *Lewis* in 1955 assumed that the shift in pH due to hypocapnia could be just as dangerous as acidosis.

In 1957 *Severinghaus* et al. defined as "normal" that ventilation "in which carbon dioxide elimination equals its rate of metabolic production as cooling progresses"; stating that "pCO_2 should be used to define normal ventilation not that pCO_2 should be constant but that it should fall as the pCO_2 does in blood cooled in vitro".

Severinghaus et al. (1957) calculated that the *same tidal volume and rate as were needed to maintain respiratory balance at normal body temperature* coincided approximately with those which would provide the above defined "normal" ventilation during hypothermia. In this condition pH would rise in vivo at the same rate as in blood cooled in vitro.

A similar approach was used by *Albers* (1962) who stated that during hypothermia better acid-base conditions could be secured if the CO_2 content of arterial blood, instead of pCO_2 or pH, was maintained constant.

Both these authors pointed out, however, that further experience was needed in order to establish if this kind of acid-base condition — which by normal temperature standards would be defined as respiratory alkalosis — was the best to ensure protection of the circulation during hypothermia.

Since 1957 many authors have pointed out that respiratory alkalosis can be the cause of metabolic acidosis both through the compensatory renal loss of bicarbonates and through tissue anoxia from vasoconstriction (*Waddell* et al., 1957; *Fairley* et al., 1957; *Eichenholz* et al., 1962; *Dobell* et al., 1960).

Acidosis following artificial hyperventilation in normothermic patients has been recognized to be mild and benign by *Papadopulos* and *Keats* (1959) and by *Robinson* (1961); spontaneous readjustment of acid-base balance seems to the rule even after many hours of hyperventilation (*Cutter* and *King*, 1961); but the question arises whether the same would be true for hypothermic patients in whom a tendency to the accumulation of acid metabolites already exists (*Bernard* et al., 1961).

On the other hand *Covino* and *Beavers* (1957) have observed that the maintenance of a normal serum pH during cooling does not prevent the five-fold decrease in ventricular fibrillary threshold associated with hypothermia.

In the last years further experimental evidence has been collected to show that myocardial irritability during hypothermia may be reduced, and the buffer base deficit in the early post-hypothermic phase may be prevented, if the blood pH is deliberately maintained at low values during hypothermia (*Manley*, 1963).

According to *Carson* and *Morris* (1962) this can be best done by adding CO_2 to the respiratory gases, inducing what at normal temperature would be a severe respiratory acidosis.

These experiences are in close agreement with the clinical observations of *Nielsen* et al. (1962) who state that the frequency of cardiac disturbances during hypothermic neuroanaesthesia is higher with controlled ventilation and much lower if the patient's respiration — with its attendant "respiratory acidosis" — is left unaided throughout the hypothermic phase.

It may be worth mentioning here that *Kolb* (1962) states that during profound hypothermia, obtained by surface cooling only, without extracorporeal circulation, cardiac action may be better protected if the expired pCO_2 is maintained throughout the procedure at 40 mmHg as in normothermia.

In practice gaseous exchanges during neuroanaesthesia with moderate hypothermia may be maintained in three different ways:

a) with spontaneous respiration, as before the introduction of the widespread use of mechanical ventilators; it is worth mentioning here that if large doses of barbiturates or narcotics are avoided, spontaneous respiration is appreciably depressed only under 30° C (*Blair* and *Fellows*, 1960; *Barila* and *Slocum*, 1955);

b) with "normal", or slightly reduced, artificial ventilation as indicated by *Severinghaus* et al. (1957), *Hebert* et al. (1957), and *Albers* (1962);

c) with artificial hyperventilation: it must be remembered here that cerebral vasoconstriction obtained through hypocapnia (*Sokoloff*, 1960; *Severinghaus*, 1960 b) is recognized to be an effective means for the reducing of intracranial pressure (*Lundberg* et al., 1959; *Lundberg*, 1960; *Bozza Marrubini* et al., 1962).

In the first chapter of this report (*Rossanda*) the actual knowledge of the relation between *the metabolic reduction* both of the brain and of the body as a whole and *the temperature level* has been summarized.

In practice it is usually assumed that for a given reduction in temperature a proportional and constant reduction of oxygen requirements is assured (*Vadot* et al., 1963).

Experimental evidence however points out that this relation is far from being constant and that wide fluctuations may occur in consequence of thermoregulation or other reflexes which may be active even at 30° C (*Gros* and *Vlahovitch*, 1957).

Moreover, individual differences in the metabolic response to hypothermia may be assumed; it follows that serial measures of oxygen consumption during the hypothermic state would be the only sure guide for cases in which total cerebral circulatory occlusion is necessary.

Unfortunately the methods at present available for measuring whole body and cerebral oxygen consumption are far too complex to be introduced in the operating room. Even the method recently described by *Engström* et al. (1961), expressly conceived for metabolic studies during anaesthesia, appears to be too slow and cumbersome for routine clinical use.

Even an approximate but simple method for the continuous assessment of the metabolic rate would, therefore, be welcome.

3. Personal Experience — Material and Methods

In the Neurosurgical Clinic of Milan University moderate hypothermia has been induced in 225 patients between December 1957 and January 1963. In all cases an intracranial surgical operation was planned.

In two cases after the induction of hypothermic anaesthesia surgery was cancelled: the first was a man with an acutely ruptured aneurysm whose neurological conditions were rapidly deteriorating, the second a young woman in whom the suspected vascular malformation could not be visualised by preoperative arteriography.

The distribution of cases by age and general and neurological conditions is shown in Fig. 2. Most cases were in the middle age group and more than one third were complicated by cardiovascular, respiratory, metabolic and/or serious neurological alterations.

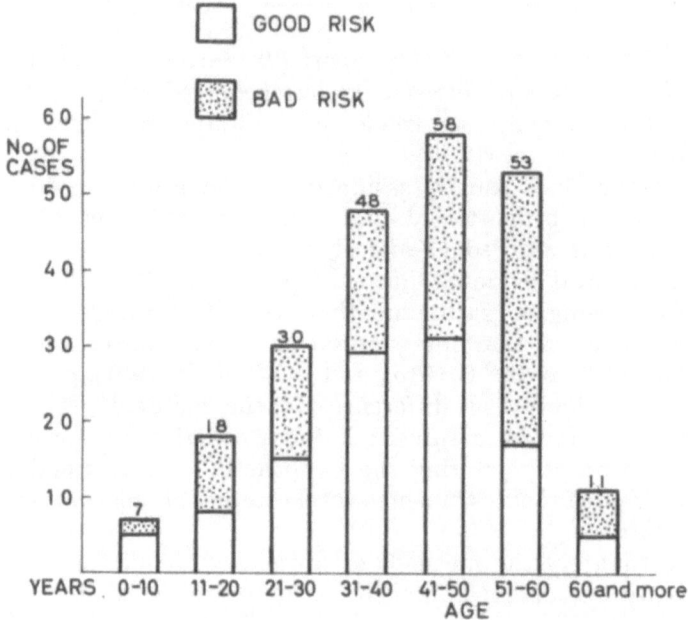

Fig. 2. Distribution of cases by age and surgical risk. Patients were classified as "bad risk" when in poor general condition, or with severe cardiovascular, respiratory or neurological alterations

In no case considered an acceptable surgical risk was hypothermic anaesthesia rejected on the basis of the above complications.

The risk for patients with cardiovascular diseases was discussed preoperatively with a cardiologist. Detailed data and conclusion on these cases are presented in the chapter of this report by *Fiorelli*.

Surgical considerations are discussed in the chapter by *Maspes* et al.

a) Cooling Methods

Between 1952 and 1958 hypothermia was occasionally induced by different cooling methods in a limited number of patients.

After a first trial with ice-bags, refrigerated rubber suits or fanning of the patient covered with a wet sheet, in 1958 a simple method based on the use of a cold air current was devised; with minor changes the same method has now been in use for nearly six years (*Bozza* and *Minoli*, 1959; *Bozza Marrubini* and *Rossanda*, 1961 and 1962).

Cooling techniques having similar features have been described by *Forrester* (1958) by *Loennecken* (1960) by *Hjorth* et al. (1962), *Vermeulen-Cranch* and *Spierdijk* (1957) by *Boeré* (1962) and by *Williams* (1962).

The method was calculated to subtract from an adult male of mean body-build about 300 calories per hour. Assuming a basal metabolic rate of about 100 cal/hour, a net subtraction of 200 calories per hour would follow: this would result in a fall of body temperature of 3° C per hour.

An essential feature of the method was the use of a fluid cooling means (air). This was in the form of a current produced by an air conditioning machine and blown on the bare body surface of the patient (Fig. 3).

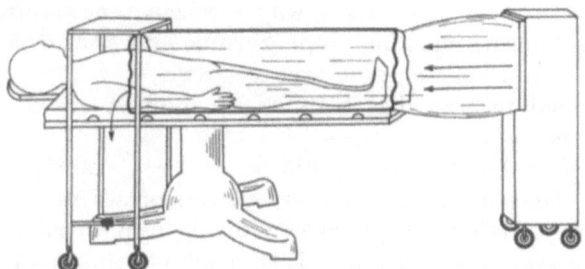

Fig. 3. Air cooling method

The air current was directed from its source to the operating table by means of a large and soft plastic tube. This was connected to a semi-rigid plastic half-tube or "tunnel" covering the patient from feet to mid-thorax. The tunnel kept the air skimming over the naked body surface of the patient; at the upper end of the plastic frame the air stream was left to disperse freely under the surgical drapes in the operating room.

The best operating conditions were obtained by keeping the air temperature between 8 and 12° C and its velocity between 0.5 and 1 meter per second. The velocity of the air current appeared of relatively greater importance than the air temperature.

No attempt was made to obtain a closed circuit of air around the patient. This was deemed to be an unnecessary complication, requiring special apparatus and care to obtain an air tight closure. Moreover, with the arrangement described an immediate and easy access to the patient was assured for the eventual treatment of cardiac arrest, for the temporary occlusion of neck arteries, for lumbar drainage of cerebrospinal fluid, for intravenous infusions, etc.; such an advantage would be completely lost with the use of a tightly closed air chamber.

The danger of a septic contamination of the surgical field was controlled both by using filtered air and blocking the surgical area with rubber sheets, double thickness blankets etc.

Technical details may be summarized as follows.

The patient was anaesthetized, intubated and positioned on the operating table as required for surgery. All monitoring devices were connected. The plastic tunnel was placed on the table and connected with the air conditioning machine as already described.

If dissection of the neck vessels was planned, the surgical field was immediately prepared and draped and operation was begun. Otherwise surgery was delayed until the temperature started dropping and the cooling rate in the individual case could be approximately evaluated. In this way a satisfactory timing between the surgical phase requiring hypothermia and the attainment of the desired temperature level was assured.

Active cooling was discontinued at about $1-2°$ C above the lowest desired level.

If necessary the final level could be adjusted exactly as required using for a time air at room temperature or warm air.

As soon as the surgical phase requiring hypothermia was concluded, rewarming was begun. Like cooling, this could proceed during the surgical manœuvres without interfering with them.

This method was used in more than 90% of the patients. In a few and selected cases two other methods were used.

Immersion in a cold water bath was adopted during the last year as an alternative to air cooling for patients expected to be "resistant" to cooling for their exceptional somatic build (obese or very sturdy individuals); the same method was sometimes used also when a low temperature level was required very early in the course of the operation, as in cases of anterior communicating artery aneurysms operated on with the *Pool* technique.

The technique adopted was exactly similar to that already described by many authors and will not be related again in detail here.

In 11 cases veno-venous cooling was employed. The method described by *Foltz* and *Frederickson* (1960) was adopted.

The extracorporeal circuit consisted of a rotary pump, of a coil made of a 5 mm. internal diameter stainless steel tubing about 1 meter long. All the apparatus had a capacity of 150 cm^3 and was primed with saline containing heparin.

The stainless steel coil was immersed in a bucket containing water and ice. The brachial and saphenous veins were dissected and cannulated with plastic catheters. Blood was sucked from the saphenous vein, pumped through the cooling coil and returned cold to the brachial vein. The pump flow was usually kept between 500 and 1000 cm^3/min.

No heparin was used except in the solution used for priming. This was necessary to prevent clotting inside the catheters during the sometimes lengthy and complex procedure of vein cannulation; as a matter of fact in females the brachial vein was often small, thin and fragile and required careful handling to effect cannulation with a catheter of satisfactory bore and to avoid rupture. During perfusion and cooling anticoagulants were not used since *Ross* (1954) and *Lelkens* (1954) stated that cold alone prolongs the clotting time enough to avoid the danger of serious embolization.

Owing to the small number of cases in which this method was used a standardized procedure was not reached.

In all cases the veins were dissected before the beginning of the cranial operation; but in some cases cannulation and cooling were postponed until the dura was open. If possible, cooling was continued until a temperature of 1—3 degrees below the final desired level was reached, as with this method an "after rise" instead of an "after drop" of the internal temperature was the rule.

At the end of cooling the extracorporeal circuit was stopped, the catheters were withdrawn and the veins ligated.

Final adjustment of the body temperature and rewarming were obtained with the air current as described above.

b) Anaesthetic Procedures

During a six years' experience on 225 patients, 23 different types of anaesthesia were used.

Only five different drugs were used as premedication, besides the routine parasympaticolythic drugs: promethazine, chlorpromazine, hydroxyzine, meperidine and hydergine.

After the first 100 cases promethazine and hydergine were rejected, since these drugs appeared to have no effect on the cooling rate.

Also for hydroxizine no effect on thermoregulation reflexes is claimed; this drug was used however in a number of cases mainly for its sedative action coupled with the absence of undesirable side effects on vital functions regulation (average adult dose: 200 mg.).

Chlorpromazine has been used routinely in the last two years: even if a significant effect of this drug on the cooling rate could not be demonstrated, a notable advantage was obtained since, after chlorpromazine premedication, the patient's internal temperature was as a rule already 1°—1.5° C lower than after any other type of premedication.

The average adult dose was 50 mg. Side effects on the cardiovascular system were usually modest and benign when the drug was used by the intramuscular route. Only in a few cases was the induction of anaesthesia in chlorpromazine premedicated patients followed by a greater cardiovascular depression than expected. Chlorpromazine was not used however in cases in which cardiovascular alterations were present before the operation.

Meperidine (50—100 mg.) was used with chlorpromazine; this was nearly the rule after the introduction of the routine use of controlled respiration with the exception of comatose, elderly or very thin patients.

Anaesthesia was always induced with a small dose of thiopentone (usually not more than 250 mg.); relaxation for tracheal intubation was obtained in nearly all cases with succinylcholine. Occasionally tubocurarine (30 mg.) with gallamine (40 mg.) was substituted for short acting muscle relaxants in cases in which controlled respiration was planned since the start of anaesthesia.

Laryngeal and tracheal topical anaesthesia was obtained with 2% lignocaine sprayed on or through the vocal cords under direct vision, or injected directly into the tracheal lumen through the cricothyroid membrane. Latex cuffed tubes, armoured with steel or nylon wire, were used for tracheal intubation.

Nearly all the available anaesthetic agents, with the exception of cyclopropane, were used for maintenance.

Some of them however, such as hydroxydione (3 cases) thiopentone and/or the so called lythic cocktails (4 cases) used alone, were rejected early in our experience as unsatisfactory from the standpoint of an adequate thermoregulation block and of a good control of vital functions balance.

The most commonly used agent for cases maintained with *spontaneous respiration* was ethyl ether, 2—3% in volume with nitrous oxide 60—70% in oxygen (about 90% of cases).

In some patients this combination gave satisfactory anaesthesia throughout the cooling procedure; but in fit adults it was fairly common to observe tachycardia or blood pressure elevations, skin vasoconstriction, muscular rigidity and sometimes even visible shivering after the oesophageal temperature had dropped by 2—3° C degrees. In this cases we tried to achieve a deeper depression of thermoregulation reflexes with the association of supplementary drugs, such as hydergine, meperidine, premethazine, chlorpromazine and their association in the so-called "cocktails lithiques".

Only in two cases was halothane alone used with spontaneous respiration for the maintenance of anaesthesia during the cooling phase. With this agent respiratory and circulatory depression appeared very early in the cooling process and further trial appeared unjustified.

Much better results were obtained with the association of ether and halothane (12 cases). These agents were used either in combination as an azeotropic mixture (two parts halothane, one part ether) or separately in alternate administration, thus taking the best possible advantages of the specific properties of each drug on vasomotor and respiratory regulation.

Ethyl ether was again the most used agent when hypothermic anaesthesia was maintained with *controlled respiration*. In these cases however muscle relaxants were commonly associated with ether so that very low concentrations (1—2%) of this agent could be used.

In the last few years the use of ethyl ether has been progressively reduced: while up to June 1962 96% of the hypothermic anaesthesias were maintained with ether, between July 1962 and December 1962 the proportion had fallen to 74%, and in the first months of 1963 has been further reduced.

Ethyl ether is still considered the safest agent available as far as side effects on the vital functions are concerned; this advantage may outweigh in many cases the risk of explosion, present even at the low concentration usually used in neuroanaesthesia.

With the broadening of experience it grew evident however that halothane, a non-explosive agent, could be a good and fairly safe substitute for ether when used with controlled respiration.

Circulatory depression appeared closely related to relative overdosage and was exceptional when concentrations lower than 1% were used. D-tubocurarine could be associated with halothane anaesthesia without untoward effects on blood pressure, provided a rapid injection of doses higher than 5 mg. was avoided; if full muscular relaxation with this drug was obtained before the beginning of halothane administration, circulatory depression was minimal or absent.

The use of halothane has been therefore extended in the last months to nearly all hypothermic anaesthesias. Ethyl ether however is still used for cases in which halothane is not well tolerated and cardiovascular insufficiency develops early in the course of cooling.

Only in half of the patients operated on under hypothermia between December 1957 and June 1962 have muscle relaxants been used during the maintenance of anaesthesia. Between July and December 1962 the proportion rose to 80% and in 1963 has reached nearly 100%.

Usually d-tubocurarine is used. In 5 cases toxiferine or allyltoxiferine have been used. With toxiferine delayed curarization has been observed in one case.

Before 1960 spontaneous respiration was maintained during the whole course of hypothermia in all patients unless a marked ventilatory insufficiency was evident. In the course of 1960 controlled respiration has been used in about 50% of cases and since 1961 controlled respiration or hyperventilation have been used as a rule from the beginning of anaesthesia, or at least during the last part of the cooling process, till the end of the operation or later.

For artificial respiration the *Engström* respirator has been used.

At present the most commonly used anaesthesia technique for a fit adult may be summarized as follows:

— the night before the operation the patient is given nembutal by mouth 100 mg. and promazine 50 mg. One hour before the scheduled anaesthesia time, chlorpromazine 50 mg., meperidine 100 mg., and scopolamine 0.4 mg., are injected by the intramuscular route;

— anaesthesia is induced with 250 mg. of thiopentone, quickly followed by succinylcholine 50—100 mg. The vocal cords and upper trachea are sprayed with 2% lignocaine solution and intubation is performed with an armoured and cuffed latex tube. At the same time the oesophageal electrode is placed;

— as soon as the effect of succinylcholine begins to disappear, profound muscle relaxation is again induced with an adequate dose of d-tubocurarine (about 30—50 mg.);

— respiration is controlled manually till intubation; next the patients is connected to the *Engström* respirator;

— once the blood pressure is stable, careful halothane induction is begun. The vapour concentration is maintained between 0.5 and 0.75% during the first phase and then reduced to 0.25%;

— cooling is begun as soon as the patient reaches a satisfactory level of anaesthesia and a stable cardiovascular balance;

— as soon as surgical manipulation requiring hypothermia is ended, rewarming is begun; anaesthesia is maintained with 60% nitrous oxide only;

— at the end of the operation, or as soon as the oesophageal temperature has reached safe levels (31—33° C) active rewarming is stopped; anaesthetic gases are discontinued and artificial respiration is maintained with air. Minute volume is carefully reduced until spontaneous respiration starts;

— as soon as adequate spontaneous respiration and protective reflexes are present, the patient is returned to the ward; if shivering occurs methylphenidate (10—20 mg.) is injected. Normal temperature is usually regained after 3—6 hours.

c) Monitoring and Biochemical Measurements

The *patient's temperature* was measured by means of electrical resistance thermometers (S.I.S., Milano), having the same features as recommended by *Stride* and *Davis* (1956), and placed in the lower third of the oesophagus, in the rectum and on the skin of a hand insulated from the cooling medium. An electrode of the same size as a *Cushing* ventricular puncture needle was used for measuring brain temperature at different depths and sites.

It was found that both during cooling and in steady state hypothermia there was a close agreement between the oesophageal and the brain temperature, the latter being usually higher by 0.5° C only.

The rhinopharyngeal temperature appeared to be a less satisfactory index of the internal and of the cerebral temperature; the temperature readings were usually 1° or 2° C lower than those of the oesophageal electrode and could be affected by vasomotor changes such as those induced by sudden haemorrhage or ganglioplegia. Wide fluctuations of the temperature of the respired gases inside the tracheal tube had no effect on the rhinopharyngeal temperature. This site of measuring was therefore used only when an oesophageal electrode could not be placed, as happened when it was necessary to induce hypothermia during the operation.

Air and water temperatures were also measured with electrical resistance thermometers (S.I.S., Milano).

Blood pressure was measured by means of a *Recklinghausen's* oscillometer on the brachial artery. In most cases at the lowest temperatures also the pulse rate and rhythm were controlled on the oscillometer.

Electrocardiographic continuous recording was used only in some of the first one hundred cases (see the chapter by *Fiorelli*).

Subsequently ECG monitoring was used only in those cases in which cardiovascular alterations had been ascertained preoperatively.

Respiratory minute volume and *tidal air* were measured in spontaneously breathing patients by means of a dry gas meter (*Parkinson* and *Cowan*) connected with the inspiratory side of a non-rebreathing system and provided with a two-way bag to assure free escape of excess gases. When artificial respiration was used, the same type of gas meter was connected with the expiratory side of the non-rebreathing system.

"Normal" respiratory minute volume to be delivered by the *Engström* respirator was calculated with the *Herzog* nomogram (*Engström* and *Herzog*, 1959).

Expired CO_2 was continuously monitored by means of an infra-red analyzer (Capnograf Godart) and recorded on a twospeed recorder (Omniascriptor Godart) (*Severinghaus*, 1960a; *Linde* and *Lurie*, 1959).

The analyzer cell of this apparatus was suspended under the surgical instrument table in order to keep it as near as possible to the patient; the cell was connected with the endotracheal tube through a 2 mm. bore, 30—40 cm. long plastic tubing; a glass tube filled with gauze was inserted half-way in this plastic tubing in order to prevent condensation water drops from entering into the analyzing cell. A tight connection with the endotracheal tube was secured by means of a latex cap covering the suction arm of the metal endotracheal connection through which the plastic tube was inserted. The measuring and recording apparatus could be removed far from the cell and out of the operating area by lengthening the connecting cable up to 4 meters. In this way accuracy and speed of response could be maintained while fragile and cumbersome apparatus could be kept out of the busy area around the operating table.

The infra-red analyzer was usually calibrated with the same mixture of anaesthetic gases used for the individual patient.

Expired pCO_2 was calculated from concentration values with correction for differences in water vapour tension at different temperatures.

The arterial pCO_2 — expired pCO_2 difference was controlled both by measuring pCO_2 in arterial blood samples and with the rebreathing method of *Campbell* and *Howell* adapted also for use with controlled respiration (*Cooper* and *Smith*, 1961; *Sykes*, 1960; *Howell*, 1962; *Campbell* and *Howell*, 1960).

Arterial blood pH and pCO_2 were measured in samples taken by means of an indwelling needle in the radial artery at the wrist. A glass electrode pH meter (S.I.S., Milano) with a thermostatic bath, and a *van Slyke* apparatus for total CO_2 were used. pH was measured anaerobically at the patient's body temperature (*Rossanda* and *Palmieri*, 1959). pCO_2 was calculated from the *Henderson Hesselbach* equation, in which the dissociation constant, pK, and the solubility factor, *a*, where corrected for temperature.

4. Personal Experience: Observations and Discussion

a) Methods

Reasons for the choice of the present anaesthetic technique among the 23 different methods tried have already been discussed in the preceding chapter.

It was soon evident however that, provided a *good block of thermoregulation reflexes without undue cardiovascular depression* was assured, nearly all types of anaesthesia could be used satisfactorily for hypothermia. This seemed however much easier to obtain, and above all to maintain evenly with volatile anaesthetic agents, than with intravenous drugs.

Intravenous phenotiazines, especially chlorpromazine, were used only in very resistant cases (about 12%). It has been observed that a dangerous cardiovascular depression (which in one of the earlier cases caused ominous cardiac arrhythmias and eventually led the patient to renal insufficiency and death) frequently developed with the intravenous administration of these powerful drugs.

Chlorpromazine was used with satisfactory results for premedication; slight hypothermia and a depression of the thermoregulation reflexes were obtained already before the start of anaesthesia, while cardiovascular lability appeared to be of minor importance.

The importance of adequate anaesthesia was more evident in the air cooling method than in immersion or veno-venous cooling. With the cold air method even a minor degree of reflex activity could be the cause of an evident slowing of the temperature fall. This can be easily explained since air cooling is much less "powerful" than immersion cooling, owing to the lower air heat transfer coefficient in comparison with the water coefficient. The introduction of curare and of controlled respiration did not appreciably improve the cooling rate with the air method; in some cases it was clearly evident that in spite of full muscular relaxation obtained with curare, thermoregulation reflexes were still active enough to hinder a regular temperature fall.

Moreover, controlled ventilation appeared to facilitate early skin vasoconstriction and therefore to handicap heat exchanges by surface cooling methods.

Cardiovascular depression, evidenced by a progressive slowing of the heart beat, by hypotension and reduction of the pulse pressure, led inevitably to a considerable slowing of the temperature fall. This could be dramatically corrected in some cases by the use of atropine and by the infusion of solutions which, at least temporarily, increased the blood volume, such as hypertonic solutions, plasma substitutes (6 or 10% dextran) or blood.

Even with an adequate thermoregulation block cooling rates differed widely for the three methods described and for different patients (Fig. 4).

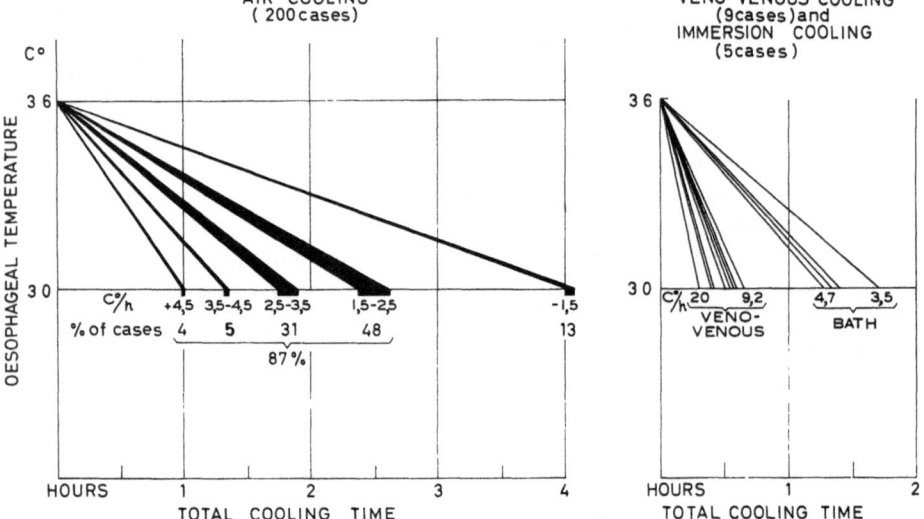

Fig. 4. Rate of body temperature drop obtained with three different cooling methods. For each method the temperature curves are schematized in order to show both the range of the cooling rates and the total time required to reach a level of 30° C of the oesophageal temperature. In the air cooling technique the percentage of cases for each cooling rate (C°/hour) is indicated

Direct blood stream cooling by the veno-venous method gave the fastest temperature falls; individual variability was much less than with other methods; air cooling was the slowest method and extreme variability among individuals was its characteristic feature; immersion cooling had an intermediate position between the two.

It may be questioned therefore why air cooling has been the method of choice for hypothermic anaesthesia in our Clinic. If we consider the additional time of anaesthesia (i. e. the time interval between the start of general anaesthesia and the beginning of surgery), required exclusively for the cooling technique (Fig. 5), air cooling, though the slowest method, was the best as far as time saving is concerned. As a matter of fact with this method anaesthesia has been prolonged in more than 70% of cases for less than half an hour besides the actual time required for surgery (Fig. 6).

This apparently paradoxical statement is explained by the fact that with the air method cooling could proceed in parallel with the preliminary surgical manipulations, such as the dissection of the arteries at the neck or the opening of the cranial dura; on the other hand both immersion cooling and venovenous cooling had necessarily to be completed *before* the start of the operation or during a pause in it, so that all the time required for these techniques was added to the surgical time. Therefore in spite of their very high cooling rate, with these methods anaesthesia was considerably prolonged.

Air cooling, however, proved to be inadequate in three different con-

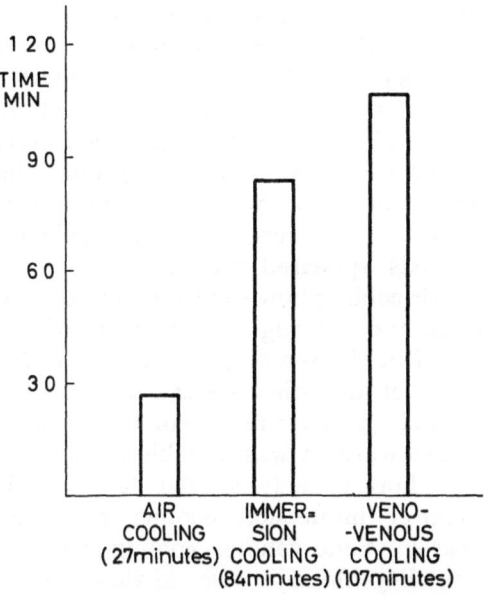

Fig. 5.   Additional anaesthesia time for cooling. Averages for the three methods

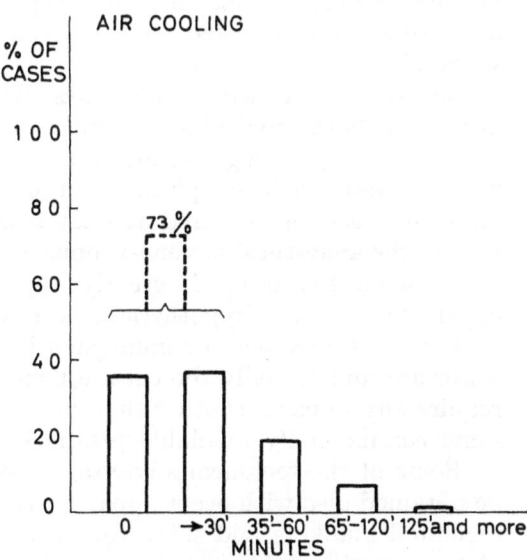

Fig. 6. Additional time of anaesthesia for *air cooling*. Percentage distribution of cases by the different time intervals

ditions: for operations on anterior communicating artery aneurysms with the *Pool* technique for which a marked degree of hypothermia (27—28° C) is required within one hour from the start of the operation; in obese, plethoric or sturdy subjects; in single individuals with high reflex activity and very labile cardiovascular balance in which optimal thermoregulation block could not be achieved without a significant degree of cardiovascular depression. In these conditions quicker and more efficient cooling methods appeared preferable.

Air cooling however had a major advantage over other methods, which far outweighed minor drawbacks; with this method *good control* of the temperature level could be assured during the whole course of anaesthesia and operation. After drop was in most cases minimal (Fig. 7); moreover by changing the air temperature from cold to warm it was possible to stop or invert the temperature fall in a short time (less than 20—30 minutes).

After immersion cooling the temperature drop was much greater. Veno-venous cooling was constantly followed by an unpredictable after rise, so that, before reaching the desired temperature level the danger zone for cardiac insufficiency and ventricular fibrillation was reached for a short time (Fig. 7). It is worth mentioning here that nearly in all cases of immersion and veno-venous cooling illustrated in Fig. 7, excessive temperature afterdrifts were checked and corrected by the use of cold or warm air.

In comparison with other methods air cooling required less personnel, both medical and auxiliary: the whole technique could be managed by a single anaesthesist with the aid, during the preliminary and conclusive phases, of a male nurse. On the other hand immersion cooling required at least two orderlies and two nurses, besides the anaesthesist; veno-venous cooling a whole surgical team.

Such an advantage is greatly appreciated in a busy surgical department, where hypothermia is a routine technique.

Cooling by ice-bags or immersion in a bath-tub filled with cold water are undoubtedly the cheapest methods. Air cooling does not require any apparatus other than an air conditioning machine and some commercially available plastic items.

Some of the technical advantages described for air cooling can be obtained also with other apparatuses such as thermostatistically regulated blankets and suits (for instance Therm-o-Rite), or complete operating tables (Auto-Hypotherm Heljestrand).

Very high initial and running costs however are a prominent feature of these apparatuses.

Whatever the method used for cooling, active rewarming was always effected with warm air.

In the first cases rewarming was continued until the oesophageal temperature had reached normal values (37—38° C). It was soon observed that even in this way shivering in the early post-anaesthetic course could not be prevented in a number of patients and hyperthermia was frequent; this technique was therefore abandoned (except in very young children) in whom prolonged hypothermia

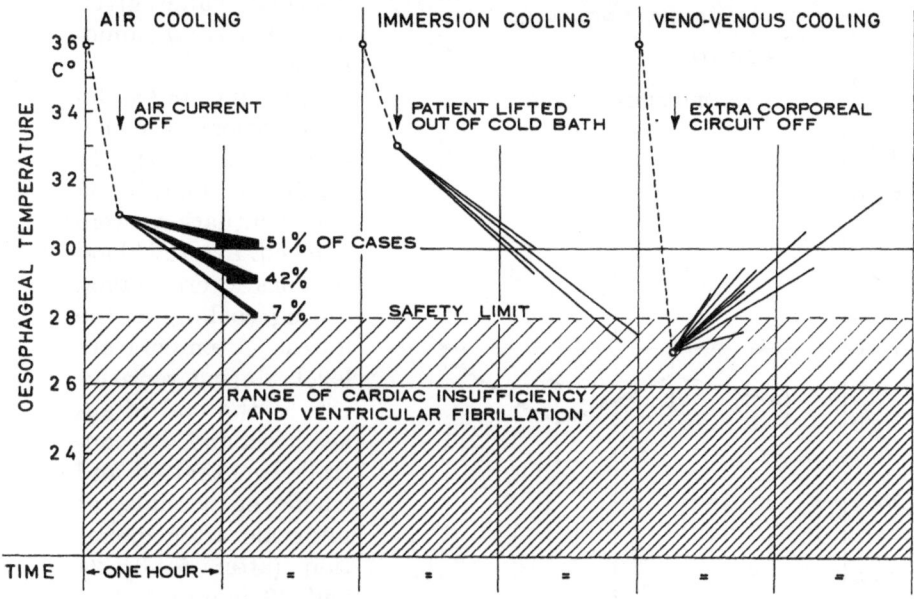

Fig. 7. Schematic representation of the behaviour of the oesophageal temperature after the end of active cooling

may be dangerous (*France*, 1957; *Calvert*, 1962; *Hackett* and *Crosby*, 1960) and patients were actively rewarmed only until safe levels of temperature (31—33° C) were reached.

Chlorpromazine, and/or the lythic cocktail, were used to prevent or treat shivering during spontaneous rewarming. This lead as a rule to delayed recovery of consciousness and cardiovascular depression. Since 1961 methylphenidate, an analeptic and awakening drug first described by *Bortoluzzi* et al. (1962 and 1963) as effective in the treatment of shivering, has been used for the same purpose with satisfactory results.

b) Respiratory and Acid-Base Regulation

Personal observations on acid-base variations occurring in spontaneously breathing patients during and after hypothermic anaesthesia have been already published elsewhere (*Bozza Marrubini* and *Rossanda*, 1962; *Formenton*, 1963). Some of these data are used in this report for comparison with observations made during and after artificial respiration.

Acid-base regulation has been studied in 41 patients. 20 cases breathed spontaneously throughout the course of hypothermia, 12 were artificially ventilated all the time with "normal" minute volumes (according to *Severinghaus*) and 9 were artificially hyperventilated with constant minute volumes 60—100% above the "normal" values given by the *Herzog* nomogram.

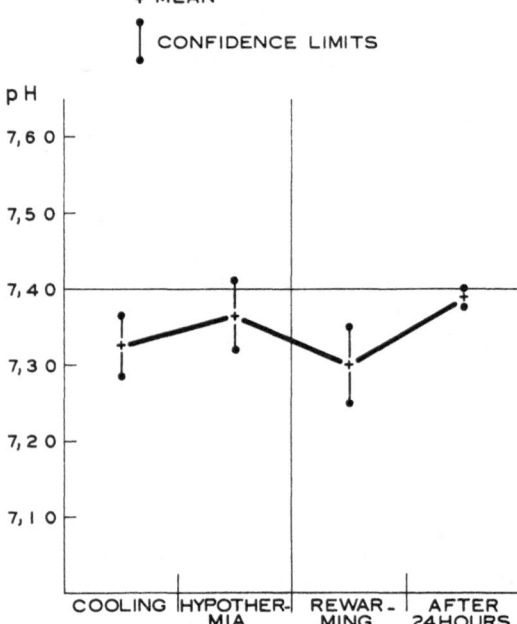

SPONTANEOUS BREATHING

+ MEAN

CONFIDENCE LIMITS

pH and pCO_2 determinations were begun as soon as steady levels of anaesthesia and ventilation were reached. Arterial blood samples were taken during cooling, at the lowest temperature level, during rewarming, at the end of anaesthesia and of controlled ventilation, and whenever possible, at intervals after operation (after 5—8, 24 and 48 hours).

Collected data are represented in Figs. 8 to 13.

Fig. 8. Arterial blood pH observed during anaesthesia, cooling, rewarming and early postoperative course in spontaneously breathing patients. Averages and confidence limits for 20 cases

Spontaneous respiration, in cases maintained with "light ether" and nitrousoxide only, was usually only moderately depressed. Minute volume at 30° C was about 30% less than at normal temperature. Wide variations from this mean value were observed in response to surgical manipulation, thermoregulation reflexes, blood pressure changes, etc.

Acid-base changes during spontaneous respiration were surprisingly small. Moderate acidosis both before, during and after hypothermia was frequent but as a rule benign and spontaneously reversible within 18 hours (Fig. 8). During the hypothermic phase slight hyperventilation and metabolic acidosis were revealed by low pCO_2 with normal or slighly elevated pH. During rewarming the usual finding was metabolic acidosis, but in a few cases this was associated also with underventilation and CO_2 retention (Fig. 9).

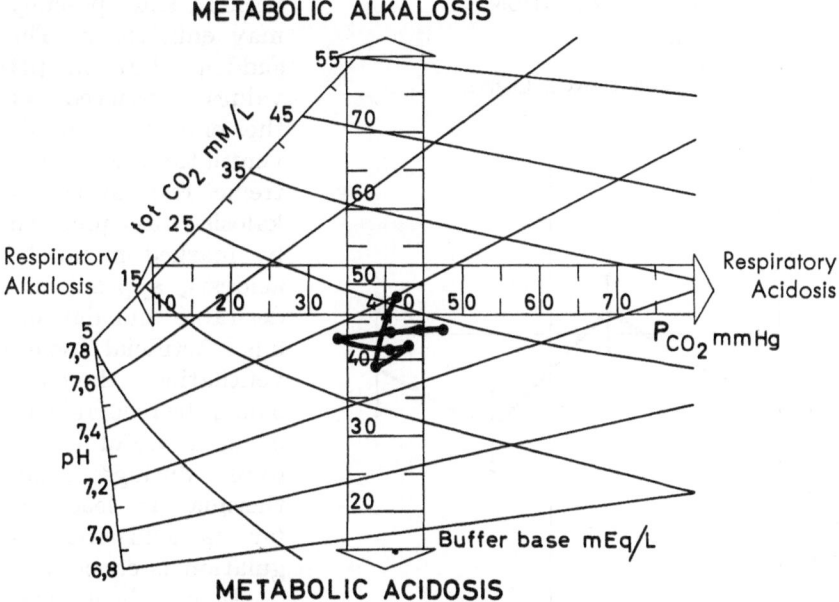

Fig. 9. Acid-base "vector" for hypothermic anaesthesia with spontaneous respiration. Averages for 20 cases. Time progression is given by arrows. First dot: anaesthesia induced, normal temperature; second, third and fourth dot: cooling phase; fifth dot: rewarming phase; sixth dot: after 5—8 hours; seventh dot: 24 hours after hypothermia

During hypothermia, *controlled ventilation* with "normal" minute volumes induced a slight alkalosis (Fig. 10). As could easily be expected the shift towards high pH values was extreme during hypothermia with *hyperventilation* (Fig. 11).

Such wide deviations of acid-base values however seemed to be far from beneficial: rewarming acidosis was clearly evident in all cases and appeared to be more marked in artificially ventilated patients than in spontaneously breathing patients.

The acid-base "vectors" (according to *Boeré*) clearly indicate that intra-anaesthetic changes in artificially ventilated patients were nearly exclusively of respiratory type; post-anaesthetic rewarming acidosis was frankly metabolic (Fig. 12 and 13).

Statistical evaluation of these data has not been attempted as the three groups of cases differed in many other features besides ventilation and were studied at different times.

It can be concluded however that intrahypothermic respiratory alkalosis induced by artificial ventilation does not prevent acidosis in the rewarming period and possibly may enhance it. The sudden shift in pH values observed at the end of artificial ventilation, when extreme respiratory alkalosis was followed by marked metabolic acidosis, appears undesirable and dangerous. Artificial hyperventilation therefore cannot be recommended as a useful procedure during hypothermia at least as far as acid-base regulation is concerned.

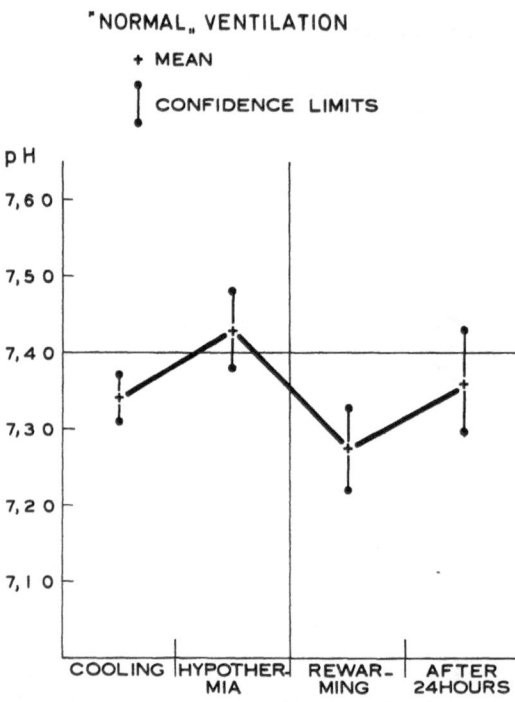

Fig. 10. Arterial blood pH observed during anaesthesia, cooling, rewarming and early postoperative course in cases artificially ventilated during anaesthesia with "normal" minute volumes. Averages and confidence limits for 12 cases

It must be emphasized however that all the acid-base alterations described disappeared spontaneously within 24—36 hours after the operation or even sooner; during this period renal insufficiency, shock or other consequences of acute decompensated acidosis were never observed.

During the first phase of artificial rewarming obtained by blowing warm air, a fall in arterial blood pressure was frequently observed; this could be prevented or treated by the infusion of 500 cm³ of blood or dextran and was ascribed to the sudden peripheral vasodilatation induced by the direct effect of heat on skin vessels. Moreover this phase often coincided with the surgical suture of the scalp; a manœuvre usually associated with considerable blood loss. However this easily controllable circulatory depression had none of the characteristics of the dramatic condition described as rewarming shock and usually associated with severe acidosis.

c) Cardiovascular Changes

Cardiac Arrhythmias

During early experience with hypothermia, when E.C.G. monitoring was a routine in all cases, it had been observed that only minor changes of cardiac rhythm were overlooked when simple clinical means of control such as palpation of the radial or brachial pulse or intermittent oscillometry were used.

Analysis of electrocardiographic changes will be found in the chapter by *Fiorelli*. In this section cardiac changes detectable by the above means only will be discussed.

Progressive slowing of the heart rate in parallel with the temperature fall was the most frequent change observed; this was noticed in more than half of the cases; in some patients the absence or disappearance of bradycardia was

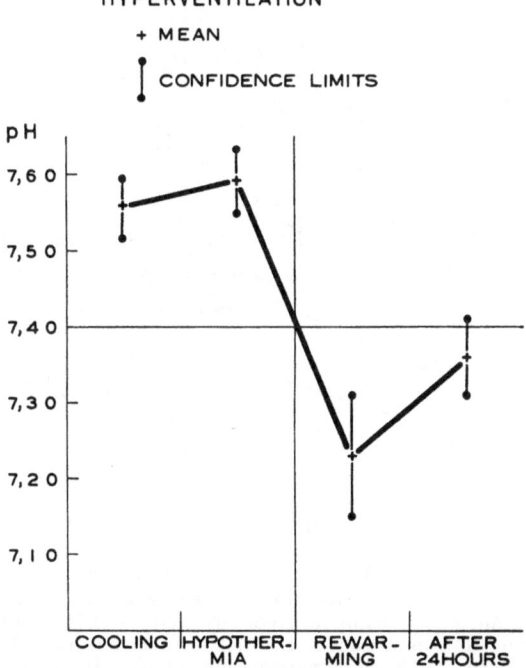

Fig. 11. Arterial blood pH observed during anaesthesia, cooling, rewarming and early postoperative course in patients artificially hyperventilated during anaesthesia. Averages and confidence limits for 9 cases

considered indicative of sympathetic activation due to insufficient depression of the thermoregulation reflexes.

Bradycardia was less frequent in chlorpromazine premedicated patients.

If untreated, this alteration of cardiac rhythm could progress to extreme values (40 or less); cardiac acceleration however could be obtained even at the lowest temperature levels (30—28° C)

7*

with intravenous atropine. The effect of atropine was unpredictable, and therefore small doses (0.25 mg.), at 5—10 minutes' intervals, were injected until the desired effect was obtained.

Cardiac arrhythmias were observed in about 14% of cases. In the first 100 cases in which hypothermia was induced up to 1960, the incidence of this alteration was lower (about 10%). Since many

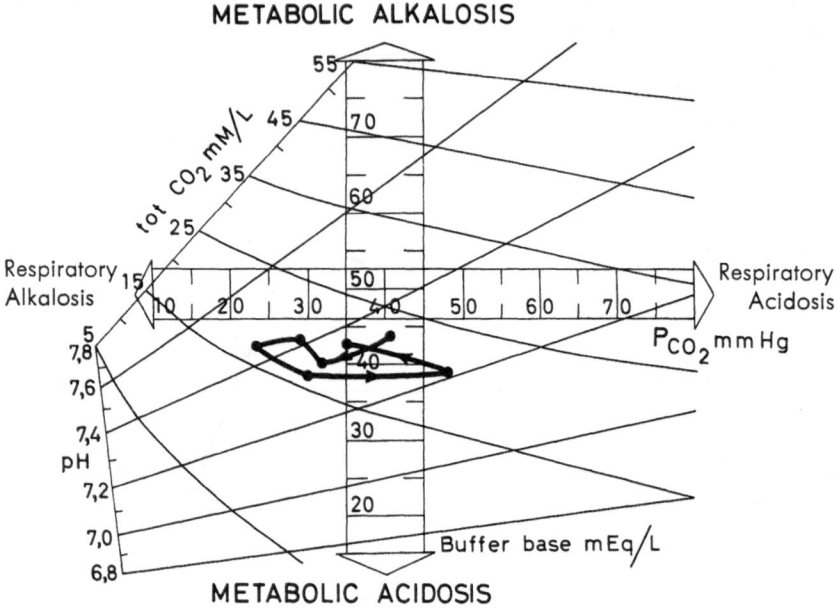

Fig. 12. Acid-base "vector" for hypothermic anaesthesia with artificial ventilation at "normal" values of minute volume. Averages for 12 cases. Time progression is given by arrows. First dot: anaesthesia and artificial ventilation induced, normothermia; second, third and fourth dot: cooling phase; fifth dot: rewarming phase, spontaneous respiration; sixth dot: after 5—8 hours, normo or hyperthermia; seventh dot: 24 hours after hypothermia

variations in the anaesthetic technique have been adopted after 1960, the possible causes of the increased frequency of this complication were investigated.

Two main factors could be evidenced: hypertonic urea infusion and hyperventilation. Table 1 indicates that the use of urea was associated with a statistically significant difference in the incidence of cardiac arrhythmias.

The slight increase observed in hyperventilated patients could very easily be due to chance (P more than 90%); on the other hand the use of urea in artificially hyperventilated hypothermic patients was associated with a marked and significant increase in the incidence of cardiac arrhythmias.

It must be remembered here that hyperventilation during hypothermia was proved to induce extreme alkalosis and a fall in the concentration of plasma potassium (*Boeré*, 1956).

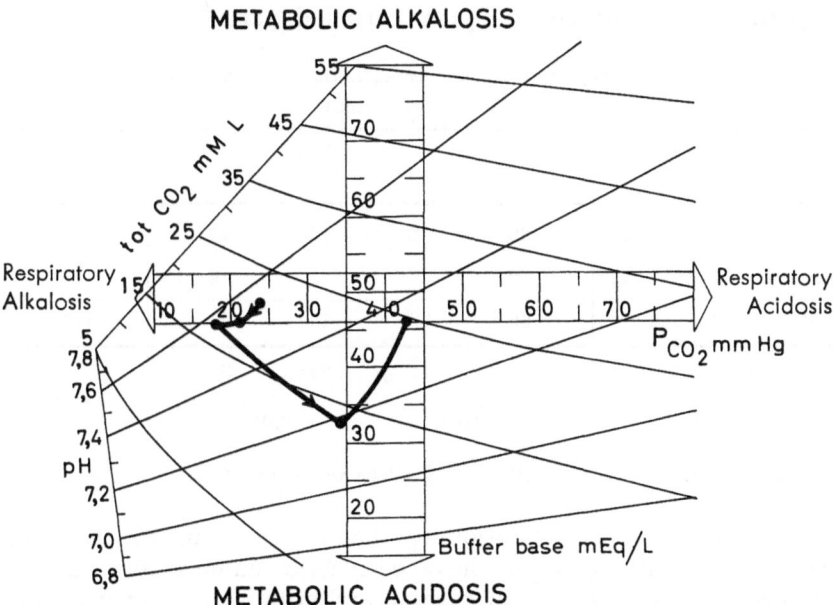

Fig. 13. Acid-base "vector" for hypothermic anaesthesia with absolute hyperventilation. Averages for 9 cases. Time progression is given by arrows. First three dots: cooling phase; fourth dot: rewarming phase, spontaneous ventilation, fifth dot: 24 hours after hypothermia

During hypertonic urea infusion an increase in expired CO_2 concentration has been observed (*Bozza Marrubini* et al., 1962), as well as an absolute increase in blood volume (*Bamforth* et al., 1962; *Alexander* et al., 1961).

In the normothermic man no significant electrolyte modification usually occurs during and after urea infusion, unless excessive dehydration is provoked (*Mason* and *Raaf*, 1961); but *Bering* and *Avman* (1960) have observed that the rapid infusion of 1.5 mg./Kg. of hypertonic urea in dogs subjected to moderate hypothermia constantly induced marked plasma electrolyte shifts and severe electrocardiographic changes. The ECG changes are believed to be closely related to poisoning by urea of the cellular sodium pump with shift of intracellular potassium; while the osmotically induced increase in blood volume is considered to be a negligible factor. As a matter of fact cardiac disturbances have been observed during anaesthesia in the uremic patient (*Compamanes* et al., 1959).

Whatever the mechanism of this effect of urea, *Bering* and *Avman*'s data, as well as our clinical observations, clearly indicate that hypertonic urea must be used with great caution during hypothermia, especially in hyperventilated patients.

Table 1. *Frequency of Cardiac Arrhythmias During Hypothermia*
Type of Treatment*

Cardiac arrhythmias	no UR NV	no UR HV	UR NV	UR HV	Total
Absent..	89	52	11	17	169
Present	9	7	3	9	28
Total	98	59	14	26	197
Frequency of arrhythmias	9%	12%	21%	35%	14%
		10%		30%	

chi square = 11,772.   P = 1⁰/₀₀ (3 degrees of freedom).

It may be worth mentioning that in cases in which other osmotically active solutions have been used, namely 50% sucrose or sorbitol, the incidence of cardiac arrhythmias remained as low as in the whole group "without urea".

Blood Pressure Changes

Severe hypotension was exceptional and was usually due to few and well identified events: sudden or profuse haemorrhage, halothane relative or absolute overdose, intravenous injection of chlorpromazine or other phenotiazine drugs or, as already described, the first phase of artificial rewarming.

Blood transfusions and reduction of anaesthetic concentration were usually quickly effective treatments in this condition; but, in isolated cases phenotiazine hypotension could only be corrected with great difficulty.

---

* UR and no UR: Patients treated (UR) or not (no UR) with hypertonic (30%) urea.

NV: Patients breathing spontaneously or artificially ventilated with "normal" (see text) minute volume.

HV: Artificially hyperventilated patients.

Pituitary-hypothalamic preoperative insufficiency due to sellar or parasellar tumors greatly increased cardiovascular lability in response to these drugs.

Intravenous chlorpromazine and related compounds were therefore used in small single doses only in fit subjects unduly "resistant" to cooling. Craniopharyngiomas, pituitary adenoma, large meningiomas of the anterior and middle cranial fossae were anyhow considered absolute contraindications to the use of these drugs.

During cooling and hypothermia a *reduction of pulse pressure*, associated with *moderate hypotension* was usually observed especially if halothane was used for maintenance.

As in the case of bradycardia, a conspicuous deviation from this rule was considered indicative of insufficient anaesthesia and of active thermoregulation reflexes.

Sudden changes in blood pressure and heart rate were frequently observed during surgical manipulation and dissection of carotid and vertebral arteries in the neck; such changes were nearly impossible to control even if deep general anaesthesia, autonomic blocking drugs and local anaesthesia infiltration were used.

d) Reduction of Metabolic Rate During Hypothermia

The metabolic rate is usually measured as O_2 consumption. CO_2 excretion cannot be used as a reliable index of metabolic rate for several reasons, the most important of which is the existence of multiple buffering systems in the body which act as CO_2 stores of high capacity (*Petersen* et al., 1958; *Farhi* et al., 1960). Rapid variations of CO_2 production and/or of ventilation are damped by these systems so that, after a rapid change, a partial equilibrium between production and excretion may be reached only after 45—50 minutes (*Glossop*, 1962; *Nunn* and *Mathews*, 1959); full equilibrium of all the buffers, as stated by *Glossop* (1962) is probably never achieved in daily life.

With progressive cooling other important changes in CO_2 excretion occur: CO_2 metabolic production is reduced, CO_2 solubility and combining power are increased.

Increases in CO_2 solubility and combining power increase CO_2 stores in the body, so that during rapid cooling, even if constant ventilation is artificially maintained, a fraction of the CO_2 produced by metabolic processes is retained in the body.

On the other hand acid-base changes, as indicated by the well-known *Henderson Hesselbach* equation, are an important cause, as well as a consequence, of variations in CO_2 excretion; it has been already pointed out that during hypothermia wide shifts, both respiratory and metabolic, in the acid-base balance may occur.

All these difficulties clearly show why an exact measure of CO_2 production is nearly impossible and would be meaningless as a measurement of the metabolic rate for usual clinical purposes.

During moderate hypothermia measures of metabolic rate however have a much narrower purpose than in other clinical conditions. Absolute and exact values are important for research work; but at the operating table all that is required is the identification of appreciable deviations from the predicted fall of the metabolic rate with reference to the temperature level; only relative values in comparison with the prehypothermic value are necessary; in neurosurgical cases moreover, plenty of time is allowed for reaching a steady state, as usually the desired temperature level is reached about one hour before partial or total cerebral ischemia is begun.

During normothermic anaesthesia with spontaneous ventilation CO_2 production and elimination have been studied by *Petersen* and *Elam* (1958) and by *Nunn* and *Mathews* (1959). It must be pointed out here that *Nunn* and *Mathews* (1959) found good agreement between CO_2 elimination, evaluated by infrared analysis, and O_2 consumption, when measurement was made after 50 minutes of a steady state of ventilation.

It was concluded, therefore, that continuous monitoring of expired CO_2 during controlled ventilation and hypothermia could be accepted as an approximate index of CO_2 metabolic production and of metabolic rate of the whole body.

The following possible sources of error were considered:

a) Respiratory quotient: this was assumed to be reasonably stable throughout the course of anaesthesia. It is realized however that very little is known about the respiratory quotient during hypothermia;

b) Respiratory variations: these were ruled out by maintaining artificial respiration with an *absolutely constant minute volume* during the whole course of hypothermia.

In a preliminary research it had been observed that, during normothermic anaesthesia, if this principle was strictly adhered to, constant expired CO_2 tensions were recorded even after many hours of anaesthesia (*Invernici*, 1962);

c) Changes in end-tidal CO_2 tension related to dead space increases: atropine, hypothermia and artificial ventilation may

increase anatomical dead space. Moreover during prolonged normo-
or hypothermic anaesthesia, with or without artificial ventilation,
appreciable increases of physiological dead space may occur owing
to changes in the ventilation-perfusion ratio of parts of the
lungs.

The absence of this important source of error was checked
by repeatedly measuring the arterial pCO_2-end-tidal pCO_2 difference; it was found that, while during spontaneous respiration wide
discrepancies between end-tidal pCO_2 and arterial pCO_2 were
frequent, so that the former could not be considered a reliable index
of arterial values, during artificial ventilation with the *Engström*
respirator a satisfactory agreement between the two values was
nearly the rule both during normo- and hypothermic anaesthesia
(*Invernici*, 1962);

d) Changes in acid-base regulation: it has already been shown
in a preceeding paragraph that during hypothermia, acid-base
variations are as a rule of respiratory type until rewarming is
begun. As a matter of fact, when artificial ventilation with "normal"
and constant minute volume was maintained, pH remained re-
markably stable near "normal" values, i. e. in the range of 7.35—
7.45;

e) Increases in CO_2 stores with the temperature fall. As already
stated this was considered to be the largest and least controllable
source of error; in hypothermia the equilibrium of tissue stores
is probably reached more slowly than during normothermia, as
since the blood flow may be greatly reduced in many tissues, as
for instance in muscles.

The temperature and metabolic fall in surface hypothermia are
however very slow processes, at least two hours being required
for a 8—10° C fall in oesophageal temperature; it could be assumed
therefore that even large errors of this type would become negligible
because sufficient time would be allowed to reach at least partial
equilibrium.

It was realized however that, on the other hand, rapid metabolic variations would result in changes in CO_2 elimination which
would bear no quantitative relation with the actual metabolic
variation.

A few examples of continuous expired CO_2 monitoring during
cooling and artificial ventilation with constant minute volume
are illustrated in Figs. 14 to 19.

A nearly linear relation between pCO_2 and oesophageal temperature was observed in all cases. Deviations from this correlation

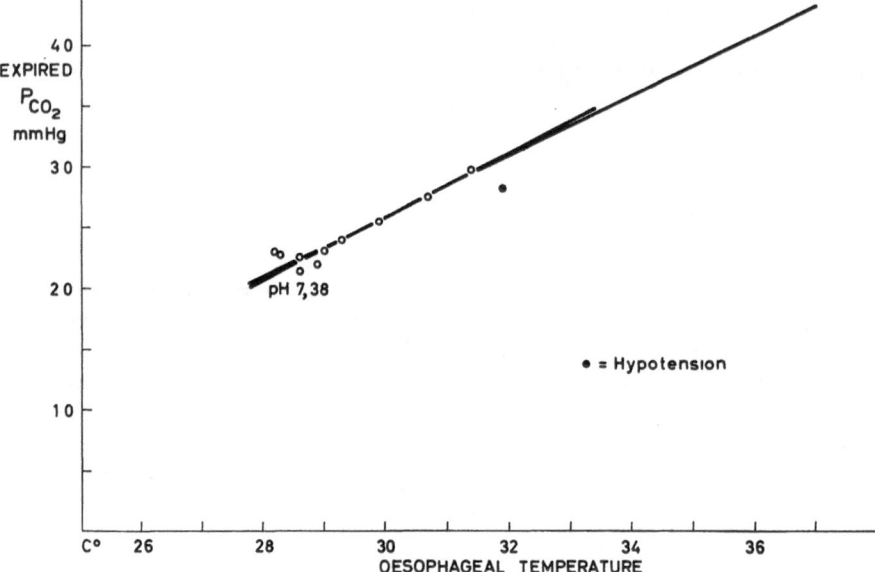

Fig. 14. Expired CO_2 tension recorded during artificial ventilation with constant minute volume at "normal" values. With the temperature drop from 36° to 28.5° C the expired CO_2 tension fell by 50%. During a brief phase of arterial hypotension a sudden and temporary drop in expired CO_2 tension was recorded

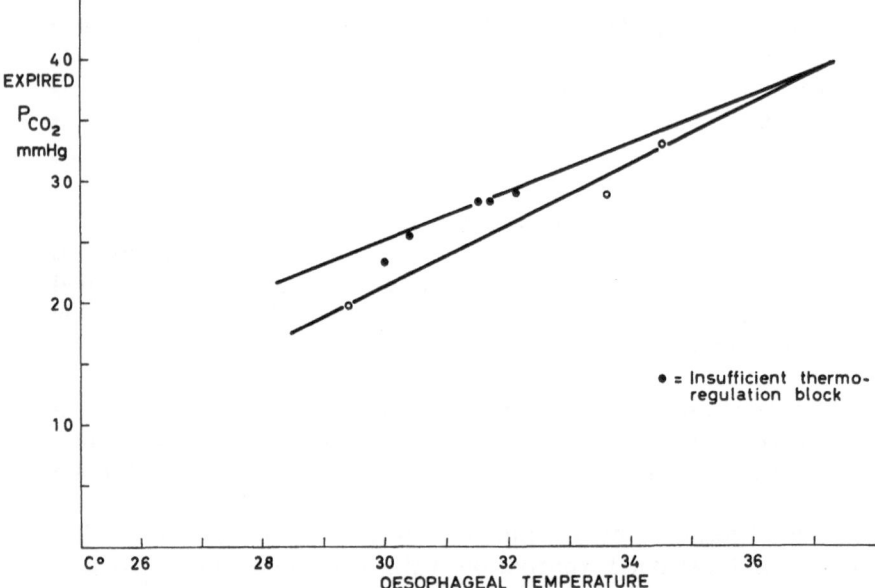

Fig. 15. Expired CO_2 tension recorded during artificial ventilation with constant minute volume at "normal" values. With the temperature drop from 37 to 29.5° C the expired CO_2 tension fell by about 49%. During a phase of active thermoregulation reflexes due to insufficient anaesthesia (black dots), the fall of the expired CO_2 tension between 37 and 30.5° C was only 38%

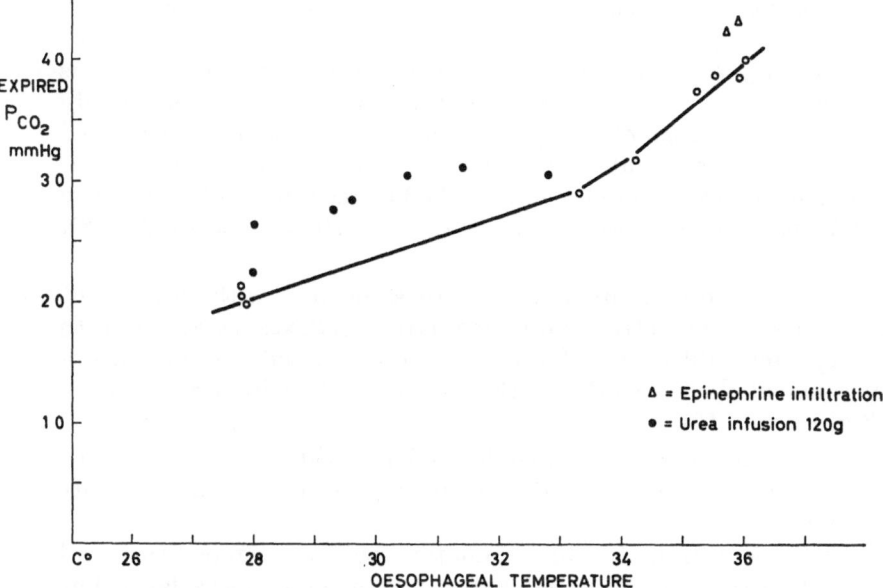

Fig. 16. Expired CO$_2$ tension recorded during artificial ventilation with constant minute volume at "normal" values. With the temperature drop from 36 to 28° C the expired CO$_2$ tension fell by 50%. Epinephrine infiltration of the scalp was accompanied by higher expired CO$_2$ tension. High values were recorded also during the infusion of a large dose of hypertonic urea

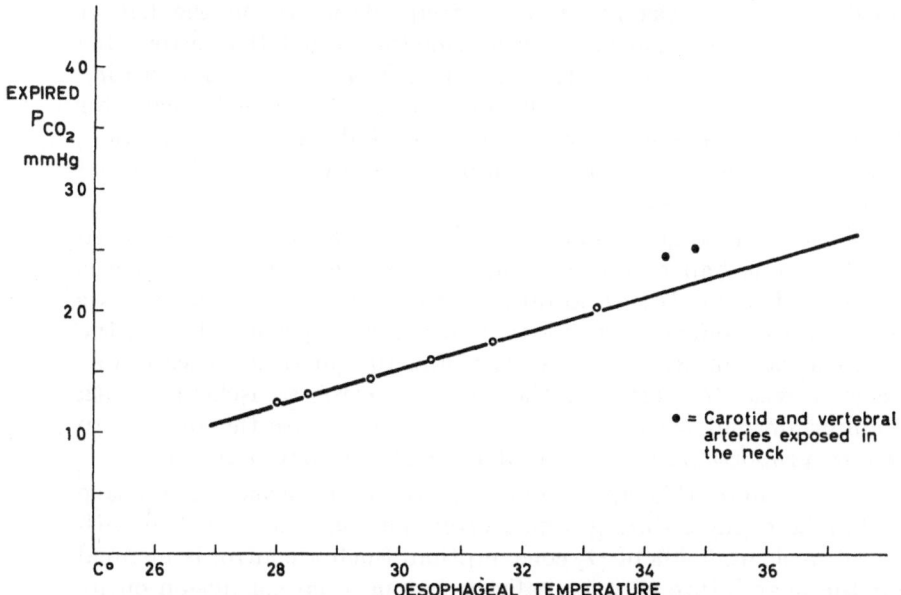

Fig. 17. Expired CO$_2$ tension recorded during artificial ventilation with constant absolute hyperventilation. With the temperature drop from 37 to 28° C the expired CO$_2$ tension fell by 52%. During surgical stimulation of carotid and vertebral arteries in the neck high expired CO$_2$ values were recorded

were clearly recognizable: sudden drops in end-tidal CO_2 were as a rule due to acute arterial hypotension (Fig. 14), as already observed by *Leigh* et al. (1957, 1961). It must be remembered here that *Gerst* et al. (1959) have observed that hypovolemic hypotension is associated with a marked increase in total respiratory dead space and consequently with an arterial end-tidal pCO_2 gradient.

Increases in CO_2 elimination were associated with insufficient anaesthesia and active thermoregulation reflexes (Fig. 15), with epinephrine infiltration of the scalp (Fig. 16), with surgical manipulation of the neck arteries (Fig. 17 and 18), with urea infusion (Fig. 16 and 19).

While the first changes could well be related with temporary metabolic activation, the effect of urea could not be satisfactorily explained.

Deviations from the linear relation between temperature and end-tidal CO_2 were more frequent at higher temperature levels but could be observed even at temperatures as low as 30° C.

Satisfactory and uneventful hypothermic anaesthesia was characterized by a regular fall in CO_2 tension. When a steady temperature level was reached, the CO_2 record remained stable until rewarming was begun (see group of circles on the left of Fig. 18); this was considered a satisfactory proof that errors due to CO_2 storage were really negligible. Expired CO_2 monitoring appeared therefore to be a useful and simple clinical means for detecting discrepancies between the expected metabolic reduction, with reference to the body temperature level, and the actual metabolic reduction.

Most authors agree that at 30° C the metabolic rate is reduced to about one half of the normothermic value; CO_2 excretion was reduced at about the same rate in most instances; in single cases however the reduction was less than could be predicted from the oesophageal temperature level (see Fig. 15); in these cases it was deemed wise to postpone the planned cerebral ischemia until equilibrium had been reached, or otherwise advise the surgeon to reduce proportionately the total time of vascular occlusion.

Up to date this approximate method of measuring relative metabolic changes during hypothermia has not been checked with direct measurements of O_2 consumption. Such a control is planned for the near future as it is realized that no final conclusion on its value can be drawn until a comparison with precise quantitative methods is made.

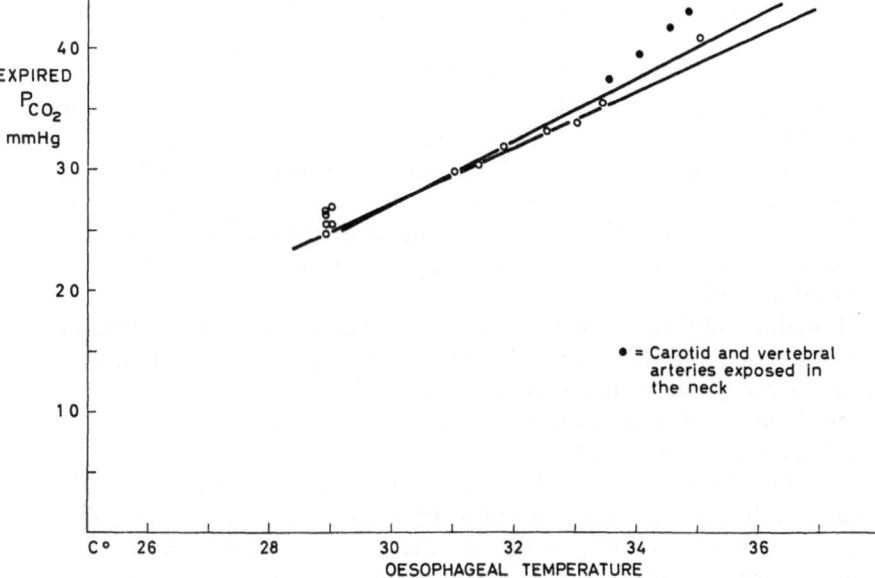

Fig. 18. Expired CO_2 tension recorded during artificial ventilation with constant minute volume at "normal" values. With the temperature drop from 35 to 29° C the expired CO_2 tension fell by 45%. During surgical stimulation of carotid and vertebral arteries in the neck high expired CO_2 tensions were recorded

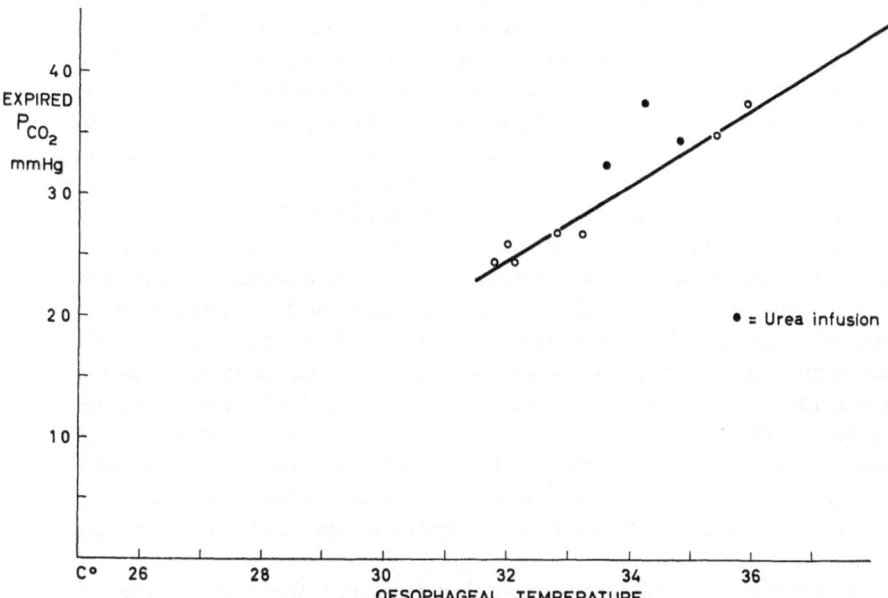

Fig. 19. Expired CO_2 tension recorded during artificial ventilation with constant minute volume at "normal" values. With the temperature drop from 37 to 32° C the expired CO_2 tension fell by 37.5%. During urea infusion high expired CO_2 values were observed

5. Conclusions

From the anaesthesiological point of view the problems of topical interest about moderate hypothermia in neurosurgery are the choice of the cooling method, the exact control of the level of body temperature, the choice of the method of anaesthesia, the prevention and the treatment of disturbances of acid-base regulation, the prediction of the maximum permissible time of cerebral ischemia.

Possible solutions for the above problems have been studied and discussed on the basis of current literature data and of the author's six years experience on 225 patients.

Surface cooling is still the simplest and safest method for hypothermia in neurosurgery.

In the Neurosurgical Clinic of the Milan University an air cooling technique has been adopted by which good control of body temperature is secured, while additional anaesthetic time for cooling, cost of equipment and auxiliary personnel requirement are reduced to a reasonable minimum well compatible with the daily routine of a busy department.

The general anaesthesia employed with this cooling method must give a full block of all manifestations of thermoregulation reflexes, both muscular, vascular and humoral. A smooth and fairly rapid temperature fall can be obtained, however, only if undue depression of circulation and heart-rate are avoided. For this reason simple general anaesthesia with curarization and halothane or ethyl ether as maintenance agents is preferred while the use of intravenous depressing drugs such as chlorpromazine is limited to occasionally "resistant" subjects.

The results of pH and pCO_2 determinations have shown that artificial hyperventilation during hypothermia did not prevent metabolic acidosis during rewarming; spontaneous respiration under light ether anaesthesia was accompanied by surprisingly narrow shifts in the acid-base balance; artificial respiration with the same minute volume which would maintain a normal pCO_2 at normal temperature, assured a nearly normal pH during hypothermia but did not prevent rewarming acidosis. Rewarming acidosis however was of moderate severity in most cases and did not give rise to undesirable clinical manifestations; in all cases a normal acid-base balance was regained spontaneously within 24 hours.

Alterations of the cardiovascular function were as a rule of minor importance, except of course when surgical emergencies such as profuse haemorrhage or trauma to vital nervous centres occurred. Cardiac arrest or fibrillation never occurred in spite of the fact that 90% of the patients were cooled to oesophageal temperatures between 30 and 27° C; bradycardia was frequently observed at lower temperatures but could be corrected with small doses of intravenous atropine.

Clinically detectable cardiac arrhythmias occurred in 14% of cases. Only in few instances did the alteration of cardiac rhythm give rise to serious concern.

A clear relation was found between the use of hypertonic urea, especially if associated with hyperventilation, and the incidence of cardiac arrhythmias.

Both this facilitating effect on cardiac arrhythmias and the above mentioned failure to prevent rewarming acidosis may suggest that artificial hyperventilation is contraindicated during hypothermia.

It must be remembered here that recent work on deep hypothermia for cardiac surgery seems to indicate that respiratory acidosis during hypothermia has a protective action on cardiac activity and helps to prevent base deficit, so that acidosis in the post-arrest and rewarming phases is reduced and quickly corrected [*Carson* and *Morris*, 1962a) and b)]. Actually in some centres no attention is any longer paid to pH during hypothermia; instead a constant arterial pCO_2 is maintained throughout the hypothermic anaesthesia (*Riabov*, 1962); this leads to extremely low pH at low temperatures, when the solubility of CO_2, and therefore the blood content, are maximal. Lower incidence of cardiac troubles and better postoperative courses are obtained (*Manley*, 1963).

Personal experience seems to confirm that in neurosurgical hypothermia also spontaneous respiration (by which a mild "acidosis" is maintained during the hypothermic phase) would be a better choice than artificial hyperventilation, at least as far as acid-base balance and cardiovascular function are concerned. Also *Nielsen* et al. (1962) after a long experience, prefer spontaneous respiration to controlled respiration for hypothermic neuroanaesthesia.

Continuous monitoring of expired CO_2 by an infrared analyzer was used as a guide in the prediction of the maximum permissible time of cerebral circulatory arrest.

If ventilation was maintained artificially with a constant minute volume, a linear relation between end-tidal pCO_2 and oesophageal temperature was found.

Among the causes of the variation of end-tidal CO_2 tension, increased solubility of CO_2 could be neglected as the temperature fall was so slow as to leave sufficient time to reach partial equilibrium. Wide differences in end-tidal-alveolar-arterial pCO_2 were ruled out by repeated controls on arterial blood and by the rebreathing method of *Campbell* and *Howell* (1960).

Expired CO_2 could therefore be accepted as an approximate guide to the reduction of relative metabolic rate induced by hypothermia and as a useful even if not quantitative monitor of sudden changes in the metabolic rate, in the acid-base balance or in the pulmonary and general circulation.

A control of the accuracy of the method is planned for the near future.

Summary

The technique of anaesthesia and the method of cooling to obtain moderate hypothermia which has been used in 225 neurosurgical patients is described. The authors favour a cooling technique using a current of air at 8°—15° C, combined with general anaesthesia using fluothane and curarization. The advantages of this method as compared with those of immersion in cold water or of an extracorporeal veno-venous circulation, consist essentially of good controllability of the required temperature, the cooling process does not prolong the duration of anaesthesia, and the method is simple.

The observed changes in the cardiovascular state, in respiration and in biochemistry are generally harmless and slight, and they recover spontaneously. It should be especially stressed that there were no cases with cardiac arrest or cardiac fibrillation. The frequency of cardiac arrhythmias was low (9%), but with the use of hypertonic urea the frequency increased significantly (21% of arrhythmias), as it also did with the simultaneous use of urea and forced hyperventilation (35% of arrhythmias). During hypothermia, hyperventilation with its resultant alkalosis seems not only unnecessary, but has the harmful effect of preventing equilibration of the acid-base balance. The continuous recording of expired CO_2, during artificial respiration with a constant volume, shows an approximate value of the reduction of metabolism as a result of hypothermia.

Zusammenfassung

Die Autoren berichten über die Technik der Anaesthesie und die Kühlmethoden, die bei 225 neurochirurgischen Patienten angewendet wurden, um eine mäßige Hypothermie durchzuführen. Sie bevorzugen eine Unterkühlungsmethode mit strömender Luft von 8° bis 15° C, verbunden mit einer Allgemeinnarkose und Fluothan und Curarisierung. Die Vorteile dieser Methode im Vergleich mit denen durch Eintauchen in kaltes Wasser oder durch extracorporale veno-venöse Zirkulation liegen sowohl in der guten Steuerbarkeit des erstrebten Temperaturbereiches wie auch in der Ersparnis an zusätzlich benötigter Narkosedauer und der Einfachheit der Durchführung.

Die beobachteten Veränderungen seitens des Herz-Kreislauf-Systems, der Atmung und der biochemischen Verhältnisse sind im allgemeinen nur gering, benigne und spontan rückbildungsfähig. Folgendes wird besonders betont: Es wurde kein Fall mit Herzstillstand oder Flimmern beobachtet; die Häufigkeit kardialer Arrhythmie lag niedrig (9%), wurde aber signifikant durch die Anwendung hypertonischer Harnstofflösung (21% Arrhythmie) oder die Kombination von Harnstoff und künstlicher Hyperventilation (35% Arrhythmie) gesteigert; die Hyperventilation mit der daraus entstehenden Alkalose während der Hypothermie erscheint nicht nur unwirksam, sondern sogar schädlich hinsichtlich des Versuches, das Auftreten von Störungen des Säure-Basen-Gleichgewichtes zu verhindern. Die fortlaufende Registrierung des ausgeatmeten CO_2 während künstlicher Beatmung mit konstantem Volumen gibt einen Annäherungswert der Stoffwechselreduktion, die durch die Hypothermie erreicht ist.

Résumé

Les auteurs décrivent les méthodes d'anésthésie et de refroidissement exercées chez 225 malades de Neurochirurgie dans le but d'une hypothermie modérée. Ils donnent la préférence à une méthode de refroidissement par un courant d'air de $8° - 15°$, combinée avec une anésthésie générale au Fluothane et Curare. Les avantages de cette méthode comparée à celles qui utilisent l'eau froide ou la circulation veino-veineuse sont le contrôle facile de la température requise, la durée réduite de la narcose et la simplicité de la réalisation.

Les modifications observées au niveau du système cardio-vasculaire, de la respiration et des relations biochimiques sont en général peu importantes, bénignes et spontanément réversibles. On insiste sur les faits suivants: pas un seul cas d'arrêt cardiaque ou de fibrillation n'a été observé; la fréquence d'arythmies était restreinte (9%), mais elle s'accrût de façon significative par l'utilisation de solutions hypertoniques d'urée (21%) ou par la combinaison de l'administration d'urée avec l'hyperventilation artificielle (35%); cette dernière, avec l'alcalose qui en résulte pendant l'hypothermie, parait exercer une influence nocive en ce qui concerne la constance de la balance acidesbases.

L'enregistrement continu du CO_2 exhalé au cours de la respiration artificielle à volume constant donne la valeur approximative de la réduction du métabolisme dûe à l'hypothermie.

Riassunto

Vengono esposte le tecniche anestesiologiche ed i metodi di raffreddamento impiegati per ottenere l'ipotermia moderata in 225 pazienti neurochirurgici. Gli autori esprimono la loro preferenza per un metodo di raffreddamento in corrente d'aria a $8° - 15°$ C, associato a anestesia generale con fluothano e curarizzazione. I vantaggi di tale metodo, confrontato a quelli per immersione in vasca d'acqua fredda o per circolazione extracorporea veno-venosa, consistono essenzialmente nella buona controllabilità del livello termico desiderato, nel risparmio di tempo addizionali di anestesia e nella semplicità di esecuzione.

Le alterazioni cardiocircolatorie, respiratorie e biochimiche osservate sono state in generale di modesta entità, benigne e spontaneamente reversibili; in particolare si sottolinea che: non si ebbero casi di arresto o fibrillazione cardiaca; la frequenza delle aritmie cardiache fu bassa (9%) ma risultò significativamente accresciuta dall'uso di urea ipertonica (21% di aritmie) o da quello contemporaneo dell'urea e dell'iperventilazione artificiale (35% di aritmie); l'iperventilazione, con conseguente alcalosi intraipotermica, apparve inutile se non addirittura dannosa agli effetti della prevenzione degli spostamenti dell'equilibrio acido-base. La registrazione continua del CO_2 espirato nei soggetti mantenuti in ventilazione artificiale a volume costante, consentì una valutazione approssimativa della riduzione metabolica data dall'ipotermia.

Resumen

Los autores relatan la tecnicâ anestesiologica y los metodos de refrigeracion que aplicaban en 225 pacientes neuroquirurgicos para efectuar una hipotermia moderada. Ellos prefieren un metodo de refrigeracion con aire corriente de $8-15^0$ junto con una anestesia general con Fluothan y curare. Law ventajas de este metodo en comparacion con la sumersion en agua fria o la circulacion veno-venosa extracorporal estan tanto en la buena dirigibilidad de las temperaturas deseadas como en el ahorro de duracion de anestesia y la simplicidad del procedimiento. Las alteraciones observadas departe del aparato cardio-circulatorio, de la respiracion y de las condiciones bioquimicas son en general pocas, benig nas y espontaneamente reversibles. Insisten en lo siguiente: No observaron ningun caso con paro cardiaco; la frecuencia de las arritmias cardiacas fue baja (9 %), pero se elevo significantemente por la aplicacion de urea hipertonica (21 % de arritmia) o por la combinacion de urea con hiperventilacion artreficial (35 % de arritmia). La hiperventilacion con la alcalosis reultante parece durante la hipotermia no solamente inefectiva, sino perjudicial respeto al intento de evitar trastornos del equilibrio acidobasico. El registro continuo del CO_2 expirado durante la respiracion arteficial con volumen constante da un dato apreciable de la reduccion metabolica obtenida por la hipotermia.

References

Adams, J. E., and *E. J. Wylie:* Value of hypothermia and arterial occlusion in the treatment of intracranial aneurysms. Surg. Gyn. Obst. *108* (1959), 631—635. — *Adams-Ray, J.:* L'hypothermie dans la chirurgie suédoise. Institut International du Froid: Annexe 1958-3 au Bulletin de L'I.I.F., 17. — *Albers, C.:* Die ventilatorische Kontrolle des Säure-Basen-Gleichgewichts in Hypothermie. Der Anaesthesist *11* (1962), 43—51. — *Alexander, S., J. C. Eaton*, and *H. J. Freedman:* Some experimental observations on the action of intravenous hypertonic urea in dogs, with particular reference to plasma volume and tissue urea changes. J. Neurol. Neurosurg. Psychiat. *24* (1961), 148—150. — *Badexer, H. S.:* As quoted in Anesthesiology *23* (1962), 887: Work capacity of the hypothermic heart. Amer. Heart J. *63* (1962), 839. — *Bamforth, B., T. J. Subitch*, and *K. L. Siebecker:* Effect of intravenously administered urea on blood volume. Anesth. Analg. *41* (1962), 46—49. — *Barila, T. G.*, and *H. C. Slocum:* Some physiological variables in hypothermia. Rocky Mountain Med. J. *52* (1955), 706—710. — *Barnard, C. N.:* Hypothermia: a method of intragastric cooling. Brit. J. Surg. *44* (1956), 296—298. — *Bayuk, A. J.*, and *C. C. Chen:* Advantages of halothane for patients undergoing hypothermia for surgery. Anesth. Analg. *40* (1961), 210—212. — *Beavers, R. G., jr.*, and *B. G. Covino:* Relationship of potassium and calcium to hypothermic ventricular fibrillation. J. Appl. Physiol. *14* (1959), 60—62. — *Bering, E. A. Jr.*, and *N. Avman:* The use of hypertonic urea solutions in hypothermia. An experimental study. J. Neurosurg. *17* (1960), 1073—1082. — *Bernard, W. F., S. E. Carroll, H. F. Schwarz*, and *R. E. Gross:* Metabolic alterations associated with profound hypothermia and extracorporeal circulation in the dog and man. J. Thoracic Cardiovasc. Surg. *42* (1961), 793—803. — *Bigelow, W. G.:* Hypothermia. Surgery *43* (1958), 683—687. — *Bigelow, W. G.:* Methods for inducing hypothermia and rewarming. Ann. New York Acad. Sci. *80* (1959), 522—532. — *Blair, E.*, and *J. Fellows:* Pulmonary ventilation in hypothermia. J. Thoracic Cardiov. Surg. *39* (1960), 305—311. — *Boba, A.:* Hypothermia for the neurosurgical patient. Springfiled, Ill., U.S.A.: C. C. Thomas. 1960. — *Boere', L. A.:* The observation of the hydrogen-ion concentration and the carbon dioxide in human blood during hypothermic anaesthesia. International Physiological Congress, Brussels (1956), 3—6. — *Boere', L. A.:* La trachéotomie post-opératoire. Presse Méd. *67* (1959), 10—11. — *Boere', L. A.:* A simple method of surface cooling. Anaesthesia, London *17* (1962), 75—76.— *Boere', L. A.:* Acid-base balance in surgery. Proceedings of the First European Congress of Anaesthesiology, Wien, Sept. 3—9, 1962; English language section 3/1—10. — *Borroni, V.:* Considerazioni sull'uso del fluotano in neuroanestesia. Anestesia e Rianimaz., Milano *3* (1962), 127—138. — *Borroni, V.*, and *M. Bozza Marrubini:* Il fluotano in neurochirurgia. Considerazioni sull'impiego del respiro controllato. Romagna Medica *16* (1962), 34—47. — *Bortoluzzi, E., R. Verlato*, and *P. Galletti:* Stato attuale delle conoscenze in tema di fisiopatologia clinica e terapia del brivido. Anestesia e Rianimaz., Milano *3* (1962), 249—266. — *Bortoluzzi, E., C. Roella, S. Longoni Bortoluzzi*, and *E. Montoli:* Methylphenidate in the treatment of shivering. Anesth. Analg. *42* (1963), 325—331. — *Bozza, M.*, and *G. C. Minoli:* Prime osservazioni su un metodo semplificato di ipotermia per interventi cranio-cerebrali. Min. Neurochirurgica *3* (1959), 168—174. — *Bozza Marrubini, M.*, and *M. Rossanda:* A simplified method for safe and controllable hypothermia in neurosurgery. Acta Neurochir., Wien, *10* (1962), 153—161. — *Bozza Marrubini, M.*, and *M. Rossanda* and coll.: Anestesia e rianimazione nella chirurgia e nella traumatologia del sistema nervoso centrale. Min. Anestesiologica *28* (1961), 365—430. — *Bozza Marrubini, M., M. Rossanda*, and *L. Tretola:* The role of artificial hyperventilation in the control of brain volume during neurosurgical operations. Symposium on Neuroanaesthesia, First European Congress of Anaesthesiology, Wien, September 3—9, 1962. Brit. J. Anaesth. in press. — *Burrows, M. M., J. W. Dundee, I. L. Francis, S. Lipton*, and *C. B. Sedzimir:* Hypothermia for neurosurgical operations. Anaesthesia, London, *11* (1956), 4—18. — *Calvert, D. G.:* Inadvertent hypothermia in paediatric surgery (and a method for its prevention). Anaesthesia, London, *17* (1962), 29—45. — *Campbell, E. J. M.*, and *J. B. L. Howell:* Simple rapid methods of estimating arterial and mixed venous pCO_2. Brit. Med. J. *I* (1960), 458—462. — *Campkin, V.*, and *J. M. Inglis:* Modern considerations in neurosurgical anaesthesia. Brit. J. Anaesth. *30* (1958), 586—589. — *Carson, S. A. A.*, and *L. E. Morris:* (a) Controlled acid-base status with cardiopulmonary bypass and hypothermia. Anesthesiology *23* (1962), 618—626. — *Carson, S. A. A.*, and *L. E. Morris:* (b) Prevention of metabolic acidosis during cardiopulmonary bypass and hypothermia. Acta Anaesthesiol. Scand., suppl. 12 (1962) 84. — *Chatas, G. J., J. D. Gottlieb*, and *R. B. Sweet:* Cardiovascular effects of d-tubocurarine during fluothane anesthesia. Anesth. Analg. *42* (1963), 65—69. — *Clutton-Brock, J.:* Some details of a technique for hypothermia.

116   M. Bozza Marrubini, A. Visca, L. Tretola, and G. Signoroni:

Brit. J. Anaesth. *31* (1959), 210—216. — *Cohen, D.*, and *V. Hercus:* Controlled hypothermia in infants and children. Brit. Med. J. *I* (1959), 1435—1439. — *Compamanes, C. J., J. W. Bellville, C. P. Boyan,* and *W. S. Howland:* Cardiac conduction disturbances during anesthesia in the uremic patient. Anesth. Analg. *38* (1959), 283—288. — *Cooper, K.*, and *D. Ross:* Hypothermia in surgical practice. London: Cassel and Co. 1960. — *Cooper, E. A.,* and *H. Smith:* Indirect estimation of arterial pCO_2. Anaesthesia, London, *16* (1961), 445—460. — *Covino, B. G.*, and *W. R. Beavers:* Effects of hypothermia on ventricular fibrillary threshold. Proc. Soc. Exper. Biol. and Med. *95* (1957), 631—634. — *Currie, T. T., N. M. Cass,* and *J. D. Hicks:* The scope of surface cooling. An experimental study using quinidine as a prophylactic against ventricular fibrillation. Anaesthesia, London, *17* (1962), 46—57. — *Cutter, J. A.*, and *B. D. King:* Spontaneous readjustment in acid-base balance at the termination of prolonged hyperventilation. Anesthesiology *22* (1961), 130—131. — *Dam, W. M.:* Künstliche Hypotonie und Hypothermie mit Halothan. Der Anaesthesist *9* (1960), 107—108. — *Delorme, E. J.:* Hypothermia. Anaesthesia, London, *11* (1956), 221—231. — *Dhruva, A. J., P. M. Javeri, G. B. Parulkar, M. M. Bhatt,* and *P. K. Sen:* Fluothane as an anaesthetic adjuvant for prevention of hypoxic brain damage. J. Exper. Med. Sci. *5* (1961), 1—7. — *Dhruva, A. J., P. M. Javeri, G. B. Parulkar,* and *P. K. Sen:* Mechanism of temperature fall during hypothermia by surface cooling. Anesth. Analg. *42* (1963), 306—315. — *Dobell, A. R. C., J. R. Gutelius,* and *D. R. Murphy:* Acidosis following respiratory alkalosis in thoracic operations with and without heart-lung bypass. J. Thoracic Cardiovasc. Surg. *39* (1960), 312—317. — *Dundee, J. W.:* A review of chlorpromazine hydrochloride. Brit. J. Anaesth. *26* (1954), 357—379. — *Dundee, J. W., P. R. Mesham,* and *W. E. B. Scott:* Chlorpromazine and the production of hypothermia. Anaesthesia, London, *9* (1954), 296—302. — *Dundee, J. W.*, and *R. King:* Clinical aspects of induced hypothermia: methods of production and indications for its use. Brit. J. Anaesth. *31* (1959), 106—133. — *Eichenholz, A., R. O. Mulhausen, W. E. Anderson,* and *F. M. McDonald:* Primary hypocapnia: a cause of metabolic acidosis. J. Appl. Physiol. *17* (1962), 283—288. — *Engström, C. G.,* and *P. Herzog:* Ventilation nomogram for practical use with the Engström respirator. Acta Chir. Scandinav. Suppl. *245* (1959), 37. — *Engström, C. G., P. Herzog,* and *O. Norlander:* A method for the continuous measurement of oxygen consumption in the presence of inert gases during controlled ventilation. Acta Anaesth. Scandinav. *5* (1961), 115—128. — *Fairley, H. B., W. G. Waddell,* and *W. G. Bigelow:* Hypothermia for cardiovascular surgery: acidosis in the rewarming period. Brit. J. Anaesth. *29* (1957), 310—318. — *Farhi, L. E.*, and *H. Rahn:* Dynamics of changes in carbon dioxide stores. Anesthesiology *21* (1960), 604—614. — *Foldes, F. F., B. Wolfson,* and *M. Sokoll:* The use of toxiferine for the production of surgical relaxation. Anesthesiology *22* (1961), 93—99. — *Foltz, E. L.*, and *E. L. Frederickson:* Veno-venous shunt for rapid hypothermia. J. Neurosurg. *17* (1960), 618—630. — *Formenton, A.:* Modificazioni dell'equilibrio acido-base e degli elettroliti plasmatici in corso di ipotermia per interventi neurochirurgici. Il Fracastoro, in press. — *Forrester, A. C.:* Hypothermia using air cooling. Anaesthesia, London, *13* (1958), 289—298. — *Forrester, A. C.*, and *J. Brown:* Prediction of oesophageal temperature in hypothermia. Anaesthesia, London, *16* (1961), 129—134. — *France, G. G.:* Hypothermia in the newborn: body temperature following anaesthesia. Brit. J. Anaesth. *29* (1957), 390—

396. — *Froese, G.:* Effect of breathing oxygen at one atmosphere in the response to cold in human subjects. J. Appl. Physiol. *13* (1958), 66—74. — *Galindo, A., J. H. Sprouse, U. Aubry,* and *M. Baldwin:* Anesthesia and ventricular fibrillation in deep hypothermia. Proc. First European Congress of Anaesthesiology, Wien, Sept. 3—9, 1962, tom. II, 140/1—4. — *Gardner, W. J., C. E. Wasmuth,* and *D. E. Hale:* Method of converting operating table into refrigerating trough. J. Neurosurg. *13* (1956), 122. — *Gerst, P.H., C. Rattenborg,* and *D. A. Holaday:* The effects of hemorrhage on pulmonary circulation and respiratory gas exchange. J. Clin. Invest. *38* (1959), 524—538. — *Glossop, M. W.:* The dynamics of buffering in man: carbon dioxide retention and release. Brit. J. Anaesth. *34* (1962), 66—73. — *Gros, C.,* and *B. Vlahovitch:* Hypothermie et ischémie encephalique. Proc. First Internat. Congress Neurol. Sciences, Brussels, 1957, Pergamon Press, 1959, vol. II, 76. — *Hackett, P. R.,* and *R. M. N. Crosby:* Some effects of inadvertent hypothermia in infant neurosurgery. Anesthesiology *21* (1960), 356—359. — *Hamilton, C. A.:* Predicting downward temperature drift during hypothermic anesthesia. Anesth. Analg. *39* (1960), 355—360. — *Hebert, C. L., J. W. Severinghaus,* and *L. R. Radigan:* Management of patient during hypothermia. Anesth. Analg. *36* (1957), 24—31. — *Hebert, C. L.,* and *J. E. Merzig:* Inflatable plastic tub for hypothermia. Anesthesiology *19* (1958), 287—289. — *Hellings, P. M.:* Controlled hypothermia. Recent developments in the use of hypothermia in neurosurgery. Brit. Med. J. *II* (1958), 346—350. — *Hewer, A. J. H.:* Deeper hypothermia by surface cooling. Anaesthesia, London, *17* (1962), 473—475. — *Hjorth, A., C. Thorsauge,* and *H. C. Berthelsen:* Hypothermia in intracranial operations. Acta Anaesthesiol. Scand. suppl. *12* (1962), 62. — *Holmdahl, M. H. son,* and *J. P. Payne:* Acid-base changes under halothane, nitrous oxide and oxygen anaesthesia during spontaneous respiration. Acta Anaesthesiol. Scand. *4* (1960), 173—180. — *Holswade, G. R.,* and *M. A. Engle:* A collapsible tub for immersion cooling on the operating table. Surg. Gyn. Obst. *106* (1958), 502—504. — *Holt, M. H., R. Benvenuto,* and *F. J. Lewis:* General hypothermia with intragastric cooling. Surg. Gyn. Obst. *107* (1958), 251—254. — *Howell, G. B. L.:* Rebreathing methods for measurement of blood CO_2 tension. Brit. J. Anaesth. *34* (1962), 617—620. — *Invernici, L.:* Utilità pratica in anestesia, in rianimazione ed in ipotermia neurochirurgica dell'analisi continua all'infrarosso del CO_2 espirato. Tesi di laurea. Clinica Neurochirurgica, Università di Milano, anno accademico 1961/62, pg. 1—63. — *Jackson, D., L. White,* and *J. H. Moyer:* Hypothermia, IV. Study of hypothermia induction time with various pharmacological agents. Proc. Soc. Exper. Biol. Med. *100* (1959), 332—335. — *Khalil, H. H.:* Hypothermia by internal cooling. Lancet *I* (1957), 185—188. — *Khalil, H. H.:* Hypothermia by internal cooling in man. Lancet *I* (1958), 1092—1094. — *Kolb, E.:* Problems of profound surface hypothermia from the clinical point of view. Proc. First European Congress of Anaesthesiology, Wien, Sept. 3—9, 1962, German Language Section 7/1—7. — *Krantz, J. C., C. S. Park, E. B. Truitt,* and *A. S. C. Ling:* Anesthesia LVII: A further study of the anesthetic properties of 1,1,1,trifluoro-2,2,bromochloroethane (Fluothane). Anesthesiology *19* (1958), 38—44. — *Leigh, M. D., L. C. Jenkins, M. K. Belton,* and *G. B. Lewis Jr.:* Continuous alveolar carbon dioxide analysis as a monitor of pulmonary blood flow. Anesthesiology *18* (1957), 878—882. — *Leigh, M. D., J. C. Jones,* and *H. L. Motley:* The expired carbon dioxide as a continuous guide of the pulmonary and circulatory

systems during anesthesia and surgery. J. Thoracic Cardiovasc. Surg. *41* (1961), 597—610. — *Lelkens, J. P. M.:* Veno-veneuze afkoeling. Acta Anaesth. Belg. *5* (1954), 69—70. — *Linde, H. W.*, and *A. A. Lurie:* Infrared analysis for carbon dioxide in respired gases containing cyclopropane and ether. Anesthesiology *20* (1959), 45—48. — *Little, D. M.:* Hypothermia. Anesthesiology *20* (1959), 842—877. — *Loennecken, S. J.:* Vereinfachte Hypothermie in der Neurochirurgie. Neuro-Chirurgie *6* (1960), 74—77. — *Lofstrom, B.:* Induced hypothermia and intravascular aggregation. Acta Anaesthesiol. Scand., suppl. III (1959), 1—19. — *Lundberg, N.:* Continuous recording and control of ventricular fluid pressure in neurosurgical practice. Acta Psychiat. Neurol. Scand., suppl. 149, *36* (1960), 1—193. — *Lundberg, N.:* Reduction of increased intracranial pressure by hyperventilation. Acta Psychiat. Neurol. Scand., suppl. 139, *34* (1959), 1—64. — *Manley, R. W.:* Personal communication (1963). — *Mason, M. S.*, and *J. Raaf:* Physiological alterations and clinical effects of urea induced diuresis. J. Neurosurg. *18* (1961), 645—653. — *Mellinger, T. J.:* Muscle relaxants and cooling rate in hypothermic anesthesia. Ann. Surg. *152* (1960), 1078—1082. — *Millet, R.*, and *D. Viale-Millet:* A propos de 42 cas d'hypothermie moyenne en neurochirurgie. Anesth. Analg. Réanim. *19* (1962), 463—473. — *Mortimer, P. L. F.:* Surface cooling. A new method. Brit. J. Anaesth. *29* (1957), 397—399. — *Niazi, S. A.*, and *F. J. Lewis:* as quoted by *D. M. Little.* Anesthesiology *20* (1959), 842—877; Effect of carbon dioxide on ventricular fibrillation and heart block during hypothermia in rats and dogs. Surg. Forum *5* (1955), 106. — *Nielsen, K. C., L. Nordström*, and *H. Silfvenius:* Hypothermia with air cooling in neurosurgical operations under ether anaesthesia. Acta Anaesthesiol. Scand., suppl. 12 (1962), 53—54. — *Nunn, J. F.*, and *R. L. Mathews:* Gaseous exchange during halothane anaesthesia. Brit. J. Anaesth. *31* (1959), 330—340. — *Oppeln-Bronikowsky, K.:* Die Anwendung eines Gummi-Skafanders bei kontrollierter Hypothermie bei 30° C. Proc. First European Congress Anaesthesiology, Wien, Sept. 3—9, 1962, tom. II, 212/1—4. — *Orton, R. H.*, and *K. N. Morris:* as quoted by *K. E. Cooper* and *K. N. Ross:* Hypothermia in surgical practice. London: Cassel & Co. 1960. Deliberate circulatory arrest. The use of halothane and heparin for direct vision intracardiac surgery. Thorax *14* (1959), 39. — *Papadopulos, C. N.*, and *A. S. Keats:* The metabolic acidosis of hyperventilation produced by controlled respiration. Anesthesiology *20* (1959), 156—161. — *Parkhouse, J.:* General anaesthesia as an aid to therapeutic hypothermia. Brit. Med. J. *II* (1957), 751. — *Petersen, P. N.*, and *J. O. Elam:* Elimination of carbon dioxide. Anesth. Analg. 37 (1958), 91—106. — *Pool, J. L.*, and *L. A. Kessler:* Mechanism and control of centrally induced cardiac irregularities during hypothermia. Part I. Clinical observations. J. Neurosurg. *15* (1958), 52—64. — *Purpura, D. P., J. L. Pool, E. M. Housepian, M. Girado, S. A. Jacobson*, and *R. J. Seymour:* Hypothermic potentiation of centrally induced cardiac irregularities. Anesthesiology *19* (1958), 27—37. — *Riabov, G. A.:* The principles of functional control in congenital heart disease in superficial and deep hypothermia. Proc. First European Congress Anaesthesiology, Wien, Sept. 3—9, 1962, tom. II, 119/1—4. — *Robinson, J. S.:* Some biochemical effects of passive hyperventilation. Brit. J. Anaesth. *33* (1961), 69—76. — *Rollason, W. N.*, and *J. M. Hough:* The influence of chlorpromazine and hydergine on pethidine and scopolamine premedication. Brit. J. Anaesth. *32* (1960), 580—581. — *Ross, D. N.:* Venous cooling. A new method of cooling the blood stream. Lancet *I* (1954), 1108—1109. — *Rossanda, M.,* and *R. Palmieri:* La determinazione del pH del sangue nella pratica clinica e nelle applicazioni all'anestesia. Min. Anestesiol. *25* (1959), 63—71. — *Sedzimir, C. B.,* and *J. W. Dundee:* Hypothermia in the treatment of cerebral tumours. J. Neurosurg. *15* (1958), 199—205. — *Sellick, B. A.:* A method of hypothermia for open heart surgery. Lancet *I* (1957), 443—446. — *Severinghaus, J. W., M. A. Stupfel,* and *A. F. Bradley:* Alveolar dead space and arterial to end-tidal carbon dioxide differences during hypothermia in dog and man. J. Appl. Physiol. *10* (1957), 349—355. — *Severinghaus, J. W.:* (a) Methods of measurement of blood and gas carbon dioxide during anesthesia. Anesthesiology *21* (1960), 717—726. — *Severinghaus, J. W.:* (b) CO_2 Spannung und Perfusion im Gewebe. Der Anaesthesist *9* (1960), 50—55. — *Sokoloff, L.:* The effects of carbon dioxide on the cerebral circulation. Anesthesiology *21* (1960), 664—673. — *Stevenson, D. E.:* Changes caused by anaesthesia in the blood electrolytes of the dog. Brit. J. Anaesth. *32* (1960), 353—363. — *Stride, S. D. K.,* and *R. W. Davis:* Thermometers for hypothermia. Lancet *II* (1956), 308—309. — *Sykes, M. K.:* Observations on a rebreathing technique for the determination of arterial pCO_2 in the apnoeic patient. Brit. J. Anaesth. *32* (1960), 256—261. — *Vadot, L.:* Hypothermie: de la physique à la physio-pathologie per-opératoire. L'Expansion Scientifique Française, Paris, 1962. — *Vadot, L., S. Estanove, R. Gounod,* and *P. Marion:* Calcul de l'arrêt circulatoire admissible en hypothermie. Anesth. Analg. Réanim. *20* (1963), 61—65. — *Vandewater, S. L., W. M. Lougheed, J. W. Scott,* and *E. H. Botterell:* Some observations with the use of hypothermia in neurosurgery. Anesth. Analg. *37* (1958), 29—36. — *Verbiest, H.:* Temperature and heat regulation. Folia Psychiat. Neurol. Neurochir. Neerl. *59* (1956), 363—407. — *Vermeulen-Cranch, D. M. E.,* and *J. Spierdijk:* A temperature controlled cabinet operating table for safe hypothermia. Brit. J. Anaesth. *29* (1957), 400—406. — *Virtue, R. W.:* Hypothermic anaesthesia. Springfield, Ill., U.S.A.: C. C. Thomas. 1955. — *Virtue, R. W.,* and *G. J. Wittenstein:* Alte und neue Wege in der Hypothermie. Der Anaesthesist *8* (1959), 285—289. — *Von Euler, C.:* Physiology and pharmacology of temperature regulation. Pharmacol. Rev. *13* (1961), 361—398. — *Waddell, W. G., H. B. Fairley,* and *W. G. Bigelow:* Improved management of clinical hypothermia based upon related biochemical studies. Ann. Surg. *146* (1957), 542—562. — *Waters, D. J.,* and *W. W. Mapleson:* Mechanism of heat loss during hypothermia induced by surface cooling. Anaesthesia, London, *16* (1961), 135—150. — *Williams, J. E.:* A wind tunnel for hypothermia. Lancet *I* (1962), 1334—1335. — *Wissler, E. H.:* Steady state temperature distribution in man. J. Appl. Physiol. *16* (1961), 734—740. — *Wyndham, C. H., N. B. Strydom, H. M. Cooke, J. S. Maritz, J. F. Morrison, P. W. Fleming,* and *J. S. Ward:* Methods of cooling subjects with hyperpyrexia. J. Appl. Physiol. *14* (1959), 771—776. — *Zaimis, E., B. Bigland, B. Goetzee,* and *J. MacLagan:* The effect of lowered muscle temperature on the action of neuromuscular blocking drugs. J. Physiol. *141* (1958), 425—434.

Clinica Neurochirurgica — Università degli Studi — Milano (Italy)

Moderate Hypothermia in Neurosurgical Operations Indications and Results

By

P. E. Maspes, F. Marossero, and G. Marini

Introduction

The use of moderate hypothermia in clinical neurosurgery was proposed on the basis of some data provided by experimental pathophysiology, such as:

1) protection of nervous system against the action of traumatizing agents,

2) reduction of the circulatory flow and brain volume,

3) reduction of CSF pressure,

4) increase of the nervous system resistance to anoxia.

Since the first application of moderate hypothermia to the human by *Fay* (1941), which is of historical value, the early papers dedicated to the use of moderate hypothermia in neurosurgery go back to 1955. Moderate hypothermia was first used for direct surgical treatment of aneurysms and the purpose was to allow the surgeon to perform temporary occlusion of the cerebral blood flow without producing irreversible damage to the nervous system. In 1955 *Lougheed* et al. published a paper on the use of hypothermia in the surgical treatment of cerebral vascular lesions. This work was followed by many others on the use of moderate hypothermia in the surgical treatment of the aneurysms such as those by: *Botterell-Lougheed* et al. (1956—1958), *Rosomoff* (1959), *Alexander* et al. (1959), *Adams* and *Wylie* (1959), *Uihlein* et al. (1960), *McKissock* et al. (1960), *Pool* (1961—1962), *Daws* (1962), *Laine* (1959), *Le Beau* (1962), *Obrador* et al. (1962).

All these authors agree on the usefulness of moderate hypothermia to allow temporary interruption of the cerebral flow, whereas enough data are not yet reported on the length of total or partial interruption of cerebral flow, which can be tolerated in the human without irreversible damage to the nervous system. The data so far acquired are based on the information given by clinical experience, since experimental data on the animal cannot be easily transposed to the human. The reasons for this are: anatomical and physiological differences in the cerebral flow, different vulnerability of the nervous system to hypoxia, other factors which can interfere with the cerebral circulation, such as alterations of the arterial walls, different innervation of the cerebral vessels, intracranial hypertension and other causes of increased resistance of the brain.

Botterell et al. (1956) state that in a middle-aged man the closure of one common carotid or of the carotid and vertebral arteries on one side should not last more than 6′ at 30° C and 8′ at 28° C. They say however that the safe limit varies from one case to another and that the best way of preventing ischemic damage should be EEG recording which could safely indicate a lengthening or shortening of the occlusion time.

Wanderwater, Lougheed et al. (1958) report routine occlusions of three or four vessels at the neck for 8′ at 28° C and for 6′ at 30° C. The occlusion of a single vessel can be tolerated without risk for 10′ at 30° C. Longer occlusions were performed in some cases: four vessels at the neck for 15′ and 10″ at the exceptional temperature of 26′ 6° C; of both carotids for 15′ at 26.5° C and of one carotid for 15′ at 31° C.

Alexander et al. (1959) report four vessel occlusions in the neck for 8′ at 31° C and intracranial occlusion of one carotid for 12′ and 14′ at 30° C without any damage.

Adams and *Wylie* (1959) report four vessel occlusions for variable periods from 4′ to 10′.

Uihlein et al. (1960) report unilateral middle cerebral and anterior cerebral artery occlusions for a period up to 24′ at 29° C without any damage.

Pool (1961) believes that occlusions of both anterior cerebral arteries for periods up to 20′ at 28—30° C can be tolerated. In 1962 he, however, warns against prolonged occlusions in elderly subjects.

Laine (1959) states that the protection given by hypothermia should not be overestimated; 3′ occlusions at 28° C could already be dangerous.

Lepoire (1962) points out the difference occurring between arteries in regards to the tolerance to temporary interruptions: the occlusion of the middle cerebral could be particularly dangerous either in normothermia or in hypothermia.

Other authors simply report the possibility of performing blood flow interruptions under moderate hypothermia without giving the number of the occluded vessels, the length of the interruption and the temperatures.

All the above authors report, together with cases in which the occlusion was well tolerated, cases of death or permanent neurological damage.

In these cases, however, the part played by vessel occlusion is difficult to evaluate because too many factors may be involved, such as: pre-operative state of the patient, the time since the last haemorrhage and complications during and after the operation. On the other hand, the fact that the majority of patients tolerated partial or total flow occlusions of a certain length at a given temperature without ill effects does not mean that this can be true in every case. Too many individual factors, difficult to evaluate in advance, can interfere in a single case. These factors can be: anatomical (variations of the Circle of Willis, collateral circulation), physiological, pathological (cerebrovascular resistance, grade of tissue oxygenation at the moment of the interruption, etc.).

According to some authors, the use of moderate hypothermia in the treatment of cerebral vascular malformations, apart from the possibility of performing temporary occlusions, can be justified by other advantages which can be provided by this method.

McKissock et al. (1960) state that in the great majority of cases of aneurysms operated on under moderate hypothermia the intracranial pressure was low, the dura was relaxed and retraction of the brain was easy even shortly after bleeding. This contrasts with what is observed in cases operated on under normothermia when associated with controlled hypotension. *Uihlein* et al. (1960) agree on the fact that moderate hypothermia provides reduction of the brain volume, of bleeding and shortens the postoperative course.

Botterell et al. (1956—1958) report that below 30° C the brain was constantly collapsed, provided that there were no large intracerebral hematomas or cerebral edema caused by cerebral hematoma or softening. In some cases there was such a reduction of the brain volume that the surgeon missed an intracerebral hematoma. According to these authors, hypothermia *per se* in ten cases allowed surgical treatment of anterior communicating aneurysms, a frontal lobectomy being necessary only once. Hypothermia, however, allows no protection against the edema which can occur during surgical operations, caused by retraction of frontal lobes or by occlusion of large veins draining to the longitudinal sinus. In three of such cases re-opening was necessary in order to resect the frontal pole because of postoperative edema. According to *Botterell* et al., hypothermia does not prevent the occurrence of intra-operative arterial spasms due to arterial vessel manipulations in the vicinity of the Circle of Willis.

Rosomoff (1959) states that the decreased mortality of aneurysms operated on under moderate hypothermia, is partially due to the better conditions of the operative field, because of reduction of the brain volume caused by the reduced cerebral flow.

Laine (1962) reports that hypothermia may prevent the arterial spasm which can occur during long and difficult dissection of anterior communicating aneurysms. He also says that the patients operated under hypothermia have a better postoperative course.

Alexander et al. (1959), on the contrary, affirm that in their cases hypothermia did not cause any alteration of bleeding or reduction of dural tension; retraction was made possible only by CSF drainage.

The association between hypothermia and osmotic agents was also studied very recently. *Rosomoff* (1961) studied the distribution of various components of the intracranial content and the modification occurring after administration of osmotic agents during hypothermia. *Bering* and *Avman* (1960) described an increased and prolonged hypotensive action of urea under hypothermia.

Most of the above mentioned authors reporting series of aneurysms operated under moderate hypothermia, state that the results regarding radical treatment and operative mortality have definitely improved. *Rosomoff* (1959), reviewing the pathophysiological and clinical aspects of moderate hypothermia, says that the reason why mortality is now reduced to 25% in aneurysm treatment is mainly due to hypothermia, thanks to the possibility of performing temporary circulatory occlusions. *Laine* (1962), *Uihlein* et al. (1960), *McKissock* et al. (1960), *Daws* (1962), *Adams* and *Wylie* (1959) agree with *Rosomoff*. *Hale* et al. (1962) and *Hamby* (1963) do not agree on the fact that hypothermia improves the surgical treatment of intracranial aneurysms.

This warning cannot be disregarded. On the other hand, from the review of the literature one cannot obtain statistical data since surgical techniques, operative indications and surgeons ability may vary.

The comparison between results obtained in series treated before the use of hypothermia in neurosurgery with series operated afterwards is of little value due to the technical improvements (i. e. the increased number of direct intracranial approaches with definitive closure of the aneurysmal sac).

Reports on the use of moderate hypothermia in the treatment of intracranial tumors are less numerous and the authors give only personal impressions on the dural tension, bleeding, operative field conditions and postoperative course, whereas statistical evaluation of clinical data is lacking.

Sedzimir and *Dundee* (1958) are among the first authors to consider the problem of the use of moderate hypothermia in the treatment of intracranial tumors and present a large number of cases. On the basis of 94 cases of intracranial tumor, they concluded that moderate hypothermia is particularly useful when associated with pharmacological hypotension in the treatment of severely bleeding tumors because the risks of hypotension are diminished by hypothermia. Furthermore, hypothermia protects the brain against hypoxia caused by retraction, decreases brain volume and CSF pressure and, in most cases, even when severe intracranial hypertension is present, allows opening of the dura without CSF drainage or the use of osmotic agents. The brain was generally shrunk and the dissection of the tumor required less manipulation and retraction than under normal anesthesia. In conclusion, according to *Sedzimir* and *Dundee*, the main advantages provided by hypothermia in the surgical treatment of intracranial tumors are: a) the possibility of performing deep safe pharmacological hypotension reducing the duration of the operation, especially in the highly vascularized tumors; b) the chances of operating with a higher precision and less surgical trauma to the surrounding nervous system and to the cerebral vessels which is followed by a reduction of intra and postoperative edema.

As for the shorter duration of the operations under hypothermia in respect to that under normothermia, it has to be pointed out that the criteria of comparison were not stated. The authors do not give precise indications on the use of hypothermia, nor any statistical evaluation of the follow-up results.

Inglis and *Turner* (1957) do not recognize any other advantage in the use of hypothermia except the possibility of performing circulatory occlusions and state that the use of hypothermia is recommended in the tumors of the hypothalamic region and in the vicinity of the brain stem, since alterations of consciousness and postoperative vegetative disturbances are often caused by these tumors. The same authors, however, agree on the fact that it would be necessary to support personal impressions with statistical data before affirming that patients operated under hypothermia have a better postoperative course. *Rosomoff* and *Ransohoff* (1960) state that the use of moderate hypothermia allowed for surgical treatment of some intracranial tumors which were beyond any surgical possibility: large gliomas of the optic nerves, craniopharyngiomas, vascular malformations of the third ventricle, etc. In these cases hypothermia improved the postoperative course while some selected patients were maintained cool during the postoperative period.

McKissock and *Taylor* (1960) in a paper on 120 cases of supratentorial meningiomas, 60 of which were operated on under normothermia and 60 under hypothermia, come to the conclusion that in most cases hypothermia improves the operative field, decreases intracranial tension and bleeding, but does not give any true advantages as far as postoperative course, neurological damage and mortality are concerned. These results are particulary interesting since they are based on a study of comparable cases for age and location of the lesion.

On the basis of eight different cerebral tumors, *Uilhein* et al. (1960), report that six were helped by hypothermia, but admit that in the case of tumors, reduction of cerebral volume was not as evident as in cases of vascular lesions, although capillary bleeding seemed less and postoperative course shorter.

As for the problem of the eventual risks from the operative use of moderate hypothermia, many authors have demonstrated experimentally that this new technique is not dangerous to the animal, and furthermore they generally agree that it produces no damage either to the human nervous system, although this has not been proved. *Boba* (1962) in a paper dedicated to this problem comes to the conclusion that hypothermia does not increase the operative risk. *Hale* et al. (1962) compare 40 cases of intracranial aneurysms operated on under hypothermia with 40 operated on under normothermia. In the former cases there was a mortality rate of 32.5% and in the latter a mortality rate of 25%. The operative risk should thus be increased by the use of moderate hypothermia. This agrees with the results reported by *Hamby* (1963).

In conclusion, the advantages of the method and its tolerability have not been controlled except for the protection against ischemic damage and the consequent possibility of performing safe temporary interruption of the cerebral flow.

On the basis of the literature and of our personal experience, we shall discuss here the following two points:

1) the indications for moderate hypothermia in neurosurgery;

2) the risk connected with the clinical use of moderate hypothermia.

Material, Methods and Results

Our material consists of 85 cases of intracranial aneurysm, 87 tumors (38 intracranial meningiomas, 14 tumors of the ponto-cerebrellar angle, 7 craniopharyngiomas, 3 pituitary adenomas, 10 gliomas, 12 arteriovenous malformations, 3 miscellaneous cases), 5 complicated carotido-carvernous shunts, 3 hemispherectomies.

These cases were operated on under moderate hypothermia between 28° C and 30° C according to the technique reported by *Bozza* et al. (1963).

Table 1. *Intracranial Aneurysms Operated on Under Moderate Hypothermia* Results in relation to preoperative conditions and type of operation

		Clipping	Trapping	Wrapping	Exploration
Group A: 41					
excellent:	34	26	8	—	—
good:	4	3	—	1	—
deaths:	3	2	—	1	—
Group B: 35					
excellent:	26	20	4	2	—
good:	2	1	—	1	—
deaths:	7	6	—	—	1
	76	58	12	5	1
Group C: 9					
excellent:	0	—	—	—	—
good:	1	1	—	—	—
deaths:	8	5	2	1	—

See in the text the explanation for Group A, B, C which represent different preoperative conditions.

Aneurysms

The aneurysms were divided into three groups: group A included 39 cases which at the moment of the operation did not show any neurological or psychiatric damage. Group B included 34 cases with various associated neurological, psychiatric or speech disturbances, with none or very little alteration of the state of consciousness without any vegetative disturbance. Group C included 9 cases, in which, besides eventual neurological and psychiatric disturbances, severe alterations of consciousness up to profound coma with decerebrate rigidity and severe vegetative damage were present; in all these last cases bleeding had occurred a few days or even a few hours before the operation.

As shown in Table No. 1, 77 out of 85 cases of intracranial aneurysm were definitively treated. By this we mean the cases in which the aneurysmal sac was ligated or trapped. Considering only 76 cases of group A and B, the results in sixty patients are excellent and 58 out of 76 cases of groups A and B underwent definitive treatment and had uneventful postoperative courses.

As shown in Table 2 we performed intraoperative total or partial *interruption of the cerebral blood flow* in 49 cases of intracranial aneurysm. All these cases underwent direct intracranial attack on the aneurysm. The circulatory occlusion was obtained by simultaneous clamping of the common carotids and vertebral arteries at the neck or by application of temporary clips on the large vessels at the cranial base. The patients' temperature during the clamping was in every case between 28° C and 30° C.

Table 2. *Cerebral Blood Flow Interruptions Under Moderate Hypothermia*
Interruptions performed: 49 cases.
Over five minutes: 34 cases.

Type		Under 5′	5′ to 10′	10′ to 15′	Over 15′
Four vessels					
at the neck:	14	8	6	—	—
One carotid:	6	1	3	—	2
Both carotids:	9	4	4	—	1
One ant. cereb.:	5	1	1	1	2
Both ant. cereb.:	12	1	1	5	5
One middle cereb.:	3	—	2	1	—
	49	15	17	7	10
An entire vascular district:	34	10	10	7	7

In 15 cases the interruption did not last more than 5 minutes. This group of patients is not considered here since occlusions of such a duration may be eventually tolerated at normal temperature. In the remaining 34 cases the interruption lasted from a minimum of 6′ to a maximum of 19 minutes. We believe that, during the time of the occlusion, in 24 of these last cases, the blood flow to the whole brain or to an entire cerebral district, was actually interrupted. These are the cases in which either both common carotids and both vertebral arteries were clamped at the neck, or temporary clips were applied on both anterior cerebrals or on the distal portion of a large cerebral artery such as the middle cerebral.

As for the duration of the occlusion these 24 cases are divided as follows: 10 cases from 5′ to 10′, 7 cases from 10′ to 15′, 7 over 15 minutes. In 7 cases (3 aneurysms of the middle cerebral, 3 of the anterior communicating and one of the posterior communicating artery), the occlusion was repeated several times during the same operation, re-occluding the same vessel, up to a maximum of 5 times, after an appropriate period of re-oxygenation. We never saw any complication from these repeated interruptions.

In none of our cases did we have any postoperative neurological or intellectual damage which could be ascribed to an hypoxic lesion.

It has to be pointed out that in some particular cases the duration of the flow interruption which was well tolerated, was actually longer than what is calculated on the basis of the experimental researches reported by *Rosomoff* (1963) on metabolism under hypothermia. According to this report the maximum period of safe occlusion at 28° C—30° C, should not last more than 10' to 12'. We can make two assumptions to explain the discrepancy between clinical and experimental data:

a) It is possible that collateral circulation pathways are available at the time of the occlusion (such as middle cerebral — anterior cerebral arteries). We actually noticed a little back bleeding in a few occasions of accidental rupture of the aneurysm during the circulatory interruption. It is also to be recalled that our four vessel occlusions at the neck, never lasted over 10' and that even the 3 cases of middle cerebral artery clamping were maintained around 10'—11'. The longest occlusions are therefore those of both anterior cerebral arteries where there is apparently greater opportunity of collateral circulation.

b) It has been reported (*Adams*, 1961) that beyond a certain duration of anoxia, an alteration of the regular cerebral metabolic pathways may take place.

Bleeding: We did not have the feeling that hypothermia substantially modified bleeding from the skin, muscles, bone and dura. We have to point out, however, that these are personal impressions not based on controlled statistical data.

Dural tension: In order to evaluate the effect of hypothermia on the brain and the dural tension, we selected only 54 cases which met the following requirements: a) homogeneous preoperative intracranial conditions with no tumors and no intracranial hypertension; b) oesophageal temperature below 32° C when the dural or brain pressures were checked; c) patients not treated with cerebral hypotensive drugs or treated only with osmotic dehydration, or with osmotic dehydration and hyperventilation before turning the flap.

The tumor and intracranial hypertension cases which met b) and c) requirements were few and thus not considered in the study.

The patients divided according to the treatment were compared with 102 homologous cases operated under normothermia.

The criteria of evaluation have been previously reported by *Bozza* et al. (1961).

As Table No. 3 shows, the mean degree of dural tension in patients under hypothermia is lower than under normothermia either in the untreated cases (2.25 vs. 2.48) or in those treated with osmotic dehydration (1.31 vs. 1.74) or with osmotic dehydration and hyper-

Table 3. *Modifications of the Dural Tension in Relation to Moderate Hypothermia*

Degree of tension	Untreated		HD		HD plus hyperventilation	
	NT	HT	NT	HT	NT	HT
Hypotension	4	4	10	11	16	16
Normotension	31	8	10	4	1	2
Moderate hypertension	17	7	2	1	1	0
Hypertension	8	1	1	0	1	0
	60	20	23	16	19	18
Mean tension	2.48	2.25	1.74	1.31	1.31	1.11

NT = normothermia.
HT = moderate hypothermia.
HD = osmotic dehydration = 30% urea, 1 — 1.5 g/Kg of body weight or 50% sorbitol or sucrose 2.5 g/Kg.

ventilation (1.11 vs. 1.31). All these differences are below the level of statistical significance, the constant lower values always encountered in the hypothermic cases are however very stimulating.

Cerebral Tumors and Other Lesions of the CNS

Moderate hypothermia was used in the surgical treatment of 87 cases of cerebral tumor (including 12 arterious-venous malformations). Considering the larger groups of tumors such as meningiomas, angle tumors, cranio-pharyngiomas and A-V malformations, we made a comparative study between cases done under hypothermia and a similar series under normothermia.

The evaluation of the dural tension in tumor cases is even more difficult that in aneurysm cases. However, the feeling is that, with a few exceptions, hypothermia did not reduce dural tension and brain volume to enable the surgeon to disregard the other routine methods of tension control. The same can be said for the bleeding:

hypothermia alone does not seem to give real advantage especially in case of highly vascularized tumors in which, during the removal of the lesion bleeding has to be reduced.

The group of meningiomas operated under hypothermia includes 38 cases (12 parasagittal, 4 of the convexity, 22 of the base). From the comparison of these cases with a similar series of 50 meningiomas operated on at normal temperature (16 parasagittal, 6 of the convexity and 28 of the base) it appears that the percentage of radical removals, of postoperative neurological damage and of death, are substantially the same. There is no difference in the postoperative course and in the length of hospitalization.

Controlled hypotension was associated with hypothermia in 16 cases of meningioma. The lowest values of maximum blood pressure were 30 to 40 mmHg for periods from 20' to 30'. In some cases hypotension was maintained for exceptionally long periods of time: in one case 50 to 60 mmHg was held for five hours.

The hemodynamic modification was generally well tolerated by the brain and the heart.

The immediate postoperative course of patients under hypothermia and hypotension was not substantially different from that of the other cases and was probably related more to the nature and location of the lesion treated and the type of the operation, than to the use of controlled hypotension.

During the stage of hypotension, the cardiac rhythm remained normal in most cases; tachycardia which normally follows the injection of gangliopegics was usually very mild.

The group of pontocerebellar-angle neurinomas included 14 cases. The result of a comparative study between homologous cases operated under normothermia and hypothermia shows that the number of radical removals, of postoperative damage and of death, was practically the same in both groups.

The group of craniopharyngiomas included seven exceptionally big tumors, four with intracranial hypertension and four with diencephalic damage. In five cases the postoperative course was excellent while a subtotal removal of the tumor was performed. All these patients were discharged without damage.

The group of A-V malformations (12 cases) was also characterized by a very pleasant postoperative course with lack of neurological damage. Hypotension was associated with hypothermia in three cases and was well tolerated.

The data coming from the study of the remaining 24 cases, including pituitary adenomas, gliomas and hemispherectomies, do not show any particular advantages from the use of hypothermia.

Inglis and *Turner* (1957), *Rosomoff* and *Ransohoff* (1960), *Uihlein* et al. (1960) state that the postoperative course of tumors operated on under hypothermia is smoother compared with the cases at normal temperature.

In order to control this statement the *postoperative course* of a particularly significant group of tumors, which includes 34 cases of basal meningiomas and angle neurinomas, was studied in detail on the base of a strictly statistical procedure. This was done to check the advantage offered by hypothermia in the treatment of cerebral tumors.

We selected two groups of 34 patients operated on for a basal meningioma or a pontocerebellar-angle tumor, one at normal temperature and the other under hypothermia.

We first compared the two groups in regard to the main factors which could interfere in the postoperative course: general and neurological conditions, complications in vital systems, nature, location and size of the tumor, etc. All these data were divided into four groups and were translated into figures. The observed differences were then analyzed by discriminant functions and results showed them to have easily arisen by chance.

Once the two operated groups, at normal temperature and under hypothermia, were found to be comparable, the postoperative courses were evaluated. The clinical observations (state of consciousness, length of the postoperative course, focal or vegetative disturbances, etc.) were translated into figures and then statistically analyzed. As the distribution of numerical values was not normal, before performing non-parametric tests, we made a preliminary comparison between the mean values using the "t" test of *Student*. The resulting difference was below the limit of significance (40 to 50% probability that the difference had arisen by chance).

Since the non-parametric tests, as that by *Wilcoxon*, increased the power of the statistical control, we thought it unnecessary to proceed with calculations.

We re-examined the observations with the method of sequential analysis. Pairs of patients were selected at random, a member of the pair operated on at normal temperature, the other under hypothermia and preference was given to the subject with a lower numerical value, which indicates a better post-operative course. The values were plotted into an *Armitage* design (*Armitage*, 1960).

This test confirmed that no difference could be detected between cases operated on under normothermia and hypothermia, at least in regards to the selected tumor cases and the criteria of clinical evaluation.

This conclusion does not imply an indication for hypothermia in the worst cerebral tumors, but gives a further proof of the tolerability of the method.

In order to study the problem of the *dangers in the use of hypothermia*, we selected only the aneurysm cases which arrived at operation in normal condition or with stable neurological or psychiatric damages. We analyzed preoperative conditions, surgical procedure concerning technical accidents, postoperative course and neurological status at the time of discharge from the hospital and at the time of the follow-up control. For this study we selected 76 cases

Table 4. *Danger Connected to Intraoperative Use of Moderate Hypothermia*
Analysis of the intra and postoperative factors which, apart from moderate hypothermia, have influenced the surgical result of the aneurysm cases.

Results	Complications				
	Operat. rupture	Definitive vessels occlusion	Recurrence of bleeding	Pulmon.	None
Group A: 41					
excellent: 34	4	2	—	—	28
good: 4	2	1	—	—	1
deaths: 3	—	2	1	—	—
Group B: 35					
excellent: 26	4	1	—	—	21
good: 2	—	1	—	—	1
deaths: 7	2	2	—	1	2

of aneurysm belonging to group A and B. In 60 of them no new neurological or psychiatric damage was found, in the postoperative course and at the follow-up control, besides those present before the operation. Six cases showed postoperative damage and ten died. The question was whether hypothermia was responsible for the damage and for the mortality. Table 4 shows that in the majority of these cases an intra or postoperative cause responsible for the damage could be detected and that hypothermia *per se* was not involved. In two out of the six cases with permanent postoperative neurological damage, the aneurysms ruptured during the operation and in two other patients major arterial vessels had to be ligated.

In two out of ten deaths, the aneurysm ruptured during operation, in four a large artery was ligated, in one there was a recurrence of the bleeding and in the last a severe postoperative pulmonary complication took place.

We could not find the responsible cause for the cerebral damage in four cases, two with permanent neurological damage and two deaths; therefore hypothermia could theoretically be considered responsible. However, even in these four cases there were enough other factors to make us believe that the damage could not be ascribed to the cooling procedure.

At any rate, the fact remains that against these four questionable cases, there are sixty patients in which hypothermia was perfectly tolerated (follow-up controls up to five years).

Regarding the risk in the use of moderate hypothermia in relation to the age and the cardiac conditions of the patients, we found in the group of aneurysms 16 patients over 50 and 18 with arterial hypertension that had excellent results (Table 5).

Table 5

Moderate Hypothermia in the Surgical Treatment of Intracranial Aneurysms Results in Relation to the Age of the Patient

Result	11 – 20	21 – 30	31 – 40	41 – 50	51 – 60	61 – 70
Excellent: 60	7	7	16	14	14	2
Poor and deaths: 16	—	2	2	6	6	—

Moderate Hypothermia in the Surgical Treatment of Intracranial Aneurysms — Results in Relation to Blood Pressure

Result	Normotension	Hypertension
Excellent: 60	42	18
Poor and deaths: 16	11	5

Conclusions

It seems from the literature, that the theoretical and experimental grounds on which the use of moderate hypothermia in neurosurgery is based, were not all verified in clinical practice. All the authors agree on the usefulness of moderate hypothermia in the protection of the nervous system against hypoxia. A certain number of neurosurgeons, therefore, perform intraoperative temporary occlusion of the cerebral flow for periods of time which at normal temperature could be sufficient to provoke irreversible neurological damage.

On the contrary, there is some disagreement on the other advantages which, on account of experimental data, should be provided by hypothermia. For example, it seems that in some cases of intracranial tumor moderate hypothermia gives an actual decrease of the CSF pressure and brain volume; but the authors reporting such advantages, actually mention only decreased dural tension and better operative fields and do not give any statistically evaluated data.

The same can be said for the intraoperative bleeding which experimentally is greatly reduced because of the decreased cerebral flow at lower temperature.

Regarding the protection against injury to the nervous system, we can say that it has not been sufficiently demonstrated in clinical practice. Many neurosurgeons however, emphasize the advantages of moderate hypothermia in the treatment of brain injuries and of some tumors, particularly those located near the brain stem, the removal of which may need prolonged retraction or direct surgical trauma to the brain stem formations.

The following conclusions reflect our personal opinion which, however, is not definitive. Direct surgery of intracranial aneurysms is the main indication for moderate hypothermia. We believe that hypothermia is here necessary in order to perform temporary intra-operative occlusions of the cerebral circulation. Even if it has been generally proved that aneurysms of the Circle of Willis can be successfully operated on without interruption of the circulation, it seems to us that nobody could deny that operating on an aneurysm at normal pressure or even under hypotension is much more difficult that when the sac is totally relaxed, because, thanks to hypothermia, the flow is interrupted.

There is no doubt that when the sac is empty, the dissection and visualization of the neck of the aneurysm is easier in a greater num-ber of cases and the ideal radical treatment can be achieved. When the flow is interrupted the intraoperative rupture of the sac is easier to avoid. This occurrence should be prevented because, when it happens, it is difficult to ligate successfully the sac without inter-rupting the flow in the adjacent vessels. If the hemorrhage is not promptly arrested, the drop in the flow can provoke severe damage, especially under hypotension, even when the ruptured sac is suc-cessfully obliterated. The accidental rupture of the sac under hypo-thermia is a minor risk because prompt occlusion of the flow enables the surgeon to dominate the situation better.

Apart from these advantages, moderate hypothermia does not give sound protection against surgical trauma and it does not im-prove the outcome in cases of aneurysm operated in coma shortly after the hemorrhage.

We cannot say that the protective effect of hypothermia on the vascular spasm induced by manipulation of the Circle of Willis is constantly present.

Regarding the use of moderate hypothermia in the surgery of

heavily vascularized tumors, or in the vicinity of the brain stem formation, on the basis of a study of two statistically comparable groups, we can say that hypothermia offers no substantial advantage either for the ultimate outcome or in the postoperative course.

We have to withold our conclusions regarding some type of tumors such as craniopharyngiomas operated on under hypothermia, because the number of operated cases is not sufficient. It has to be said, however, that hypothermia seems to provide protection against the endocrine and metabolic postoperative disorders.

Hypothermia is furthermore indicated in some cases of A-V malformations, the treatment of which may be facilitated by the interruption of the blood flow.

From our study we deduce that other surgical advantages eventually offered by hypothermia such as decreased dural tension, decreased blood flow, bleeding and brain volume reduction, are present but irrelevant, and do not justify the use of hypothermia, because they are more easily obtained by other means.

From a statistical evaluation of a group of aneurysms, we can conclude that, if correctly carried out, moderate hypothermia does not imply any special risk, even in old and hypertensive patients.

Summary

On the basis of the data of the literature and from the experience of 180 personal cases, the Authors discuss the indications, advantages and risks connected with the use of moderate hypothermia in clinical neurosurgery

Fundamental indication is direct intracranial attack in the surgery of intracranial aneurysms, in order to allow temporary interruption of cerebral flow for periods of time which would not be tolerated at normal temperature.

From a comparison between a group of patients with intracranial tumors operated on under hypothermia and another similar group operated on at normal temperature, it seems that hypothermia does not offer substantial advantages except in cases of tumor in the vicinity of midline structures.

Other reported effects of hypothermia, such as reduction of dural tension, of brain volume and bleeding, are present but irrelevant and do not justify the use of hypothermia because they are more easily obtained by other means.

From a statistical evaluation of a group of patients with intracranial aneurysms, it appears that moderate hypothermia, if correctly carried out, does not imply any special risk, even in old and hypertensive patients.

136 P. E. Maspes, F. Marossero, and G. Marini:

Zusammenfassung

An Hand der Angaben der Literatur und der Erfahrungen bei 180 eigenen Fällen besprechen die Autoren die Indikationen, Vorteile und Gefahren, die sich aus der Anwendung der mäßigen Hypothermie in der Neurochirurgie ergeben.

Hauptindikation ist das direkte operative Angehen intrakranieller Aneurysmen, um eine vorübergehende Unterbrechung der zerebralen Zirkulation für längere Zeitspannen zu ermöglichen, als bei normaler Temperatur vertragen wird.

Ein Vergleich von Patientengruppen mit intrakraniellen Tumoren, die unter Hypothermie operiert wurden, mit entsprechenden Gruppen, die bei normaler Temperatur operiert worden sind, hat ergeben, daß die Hypothermie keine sicheren Vorteile bietet, abgesehen von Tumoren in der Nähe der Mittellinienstrukturen.

Andere der Hypothermie zugeschriebene Wirkungen, wie Verminderung der Spannung des Duralsackes, des Hirnvolumens und der intraoperativen Blutungsneigung, sind zwar vorhanden, aber nicht so gewichtig, daß deshalb die Anwendung der Hypothermie gerechtfertigt wäre, weil sie auf andere Weise leichter zu erreichen sind.

Aus einer statistischen Analyse einer Gruppe von Patienten mit intrakraniellen Aneurysmen geht hervor, daß die mäßige Hypothermie, wenn sie richtig ausgeführt wird, kein besonderes Risiko bedeutet, selbst nicht bei älteren Patienten oder Hypertonikern.

Résumé

D'après les cas déjà connus et décrits en littérature médicale et d'après l'expérience de 180 cas personnels, les auteurs analysent les indications, avantages et risques de l'emploi de l'hypothermie modérée en neurochirurgie.

L'indication fondamentale en est l'accès intracranien direct dans la chirurgie des anevrismes intracraniens, afin de permettre l'interruption temporaire de l'irrigation cérébrale pendant un certain laps de temps, ce qui ne serait pas toléré à une température normale. D'après comparaison entre un groupe de malades présentant des tumeurs intracraniennes opérés sous hypothermie et un groupe similaire opérés à température normale, il semble que l'hypothermie n'offre pas d'avantages substantiels, excepté dans les cas de tumeurs situées dans le voisinage des structures médianes.

D'autres résultats de l'hypothermie, tels que la réduction de la tension durale, réduction du volume du cerveau et du saignement, sont réels, mais ne justifient pas l'emploi de l'hypothermie car ces résultats peuvent être plus facilement obtenus par d'autres moyens.

D'après une évaluation statistique d'un groupe de malades présentant des anevrismes intracraniens il résulte que l'hypothermie modérée, si elle est correctement conduite, n'implique aucun risque spécial même sur des malades âgés et hypertendus.

Riassunto

In base ai dati riportati dalla letteratura ed alla personale esperienza costituita da 180 casi, gli autori discutono le indicazioni, i vantaggi ed i rischi connessi con l'impiego clinico dell'ipotermia moderata in neurochirurgia.

L'indicazione fondamentale è costituita dall'attacco diretto intracranico nella chirurgia degli aneurismi endocranici, allo scopo di permettere la sospensione temporanea del circolo cerebrale per una durata di tempo non tollerabile in normotermia.

Dal paragone tra un gruppo di pazienti portatori di tumori endocranici operati in ipotermia ed un gruppo omologo operato in normotermia, non sembra che l'ipotermia offra sostanziali vantaggi eccetto quando si tratti di tumori in prossimità delle strutture della linea mediana.

Altri vantaggi, quali la riduzione della tensione durale, del flusso ematico cerebrale, del sanguinamento e del volume encefalico, sono presenti ma non tanto rilevanti da giustificare di per sè l'impiego dell'ipotermia moderata, essendo più facilmente ottenuti con altri mezzi.

Da uno studio statistico condotto su di un gruppo di pazienti portatori di aneurismi endocranici, non sembra che l'ipotermia moderata, se correttamente impiegata, implichi rischi particolari, anche in soggetti anziani ed ipertesi arteriosi.

Resumen

Basandose en los casos ya conocidos y descritos en la literatura médica y en 180 casos personales los autores analizan las indicaciones, ventajas y riesgos del empleo de la hipotermia moderada en neurocirugía.

Su indicación fundamental es para el abordaje intracraneal directo de los aneurismas, con el fin de permitir la interrupción temporal de la irrigación cerebral durante un lapso de tiempo, que no sería tolerado a una temperatura normal. Según los estudios comparativos entre un grupo de enfermos con tumores intracraneales operados bajo hipotermia y un grupo similar operado que la temperatura normal parece ser que la hipotermia no ofrece ventajas evidentes, excepto en los casos de tumores situados en las cercanias de estructuras mediales.

Otros resultados de la hipotermia, tales como la redución de la tensión dural, reducción del volumen cerebral y de la hemorragia son evidentes, pero no justifican el empleo de la hipotermia porque estos resultados pueden obtenerse facilmente por otros medios.

Según una valoración estadística de un grupo de enfermos con aneurismas intracraneales resulta que la hipotermia moderada, si se lleva a cabo correctamente, no implica ningún riesgo especial incluso para los enfermos de edad avanzada e hipotensos.

References

Adams, J. E., and *E. J. Wylie:* Value of hypothermia and arterial occlusion in the treatment of intracranial aneurysms. Surg. Gyn. Obst. *108* (1959), 631—635. — *Adams, J. E.:* Cerebral metabolic studies on the human during total cerebral arterial occlusion and hypothermia. J. Neurosurg. *18* (1961), 168—174. — *Alexander, E., C. H. Davis*, and *N. K. Kester:* Intracranial aneurysms: Methods of treatment: Value of hypothermia in the surgical approach. A.M.A. Arch. Neurol. Psychiat. *81* (1959), 684—692. — *Armitage, P.:* Sequential medical trials. Oxford: Blackwell Scientific Publication. 1960. — *Bering, E. A.*, and *N. Avman:* The use of hypertonic urea solutions in Hypothermia. J. Neurosurg. *17* (1960), 1073—1082. — *Boba, A.:* Hypothermia. Appraisal of risk in 110 consecutive patients. J. Neurosurg. *19* (1962), 924—933. — *Botterell, E. H., W. M. Lougheed, J. W. Scott*, and *S. L. Vandewater:* Hypothermia and interruption of carotid or carotid and vertebral circulation in the surgical management of intracranial aneurysms. J. Neurosurg. *13* (1956), 1—42. — *Botterell, E. H., W. M. Lougheed, T. P. Morley*, and *S. L. Vandewater:* Hypothermia in the surgical treatment of ruptured intracranial aneurysms. J. Neurosurg. *15* (1958), 4—18. — *Bozza, M. L., P. E. Maspes*, and *M. Rossanda:* The control of brain volume and tension during intracranial operation. Brit. J. Anaesthesia *33* (1961), 132—

146. — *Bozza, M. L., A. Visca, L. Tretola,* and *G. Signoroni:* Methods of moderate hypothermia in neuroanaesthesia. Clinical observations on physiological and metabolic changes. Acta Neurochirurgica, Suppl. XIII. Hypothermia in Neurosurgery. Wien: Springer. 1964. — *Daws Alex, R.:* Surgical treatment of intracranial aneurysms under hypothermia and controlled respiration. J. Neurol. Neurosurg. Psychiat. *25* (1962), 394. — *Fay, T.:* Clinical report and evaluation of low temperature in treatment of cancer. Proc. Interstate Post-grad M.A. North America (1941), p. 292—297. — *Hale, D. E., J. S. Collis,* and *M. K. King:* Intracranial aneurysmal surgery with and without hypothermia. Surgery *52* (1962), 338—341. —*Hamby, W.:* Intracranial surgery for aneurysms. Effect of hypothermia upon survival. J. Neurosurg. *20* (1963), 41—45. — *Inglis, J. M.,* and *E. Turner:* Use of hypothermia in non vascular intracranial tumors. Brit. Med. J. *1* (1957), 1335—1337. — *Laine, E.:* Traitment chirurgical des anéurysmes de l'artère communicante antérieure. I° Congres Européen de Neurochirurgie. Zurich, 16—19 Jullet 1959, pp. 131—132. Paris: Masson et Cie. — *Laine, E.:* L'hypothermie en neurochirurgie, pp. 25—33. Paris: Masson et Cie. 1963. — *Le Beau, J.:* Anéurysmes de l'artère communicante antérieure, ruptures et indications neurochirurgicales. Neurochirurgia *5* (1962), 38—57. — *Lepoire, J.:* L'Hypothermie en neurochirurgie, p. 36. Paris: Masson et Cie. 1963. — *Lougheed, W. M., W. H. Sweet, J. C. White,* and *W. R. Brewster:* The use of hypothermia in surgical treatment of cerebral vascular lesions. J. Neurosurg. *12* (1955), 240—255. — *McKissock, W.,* and *J. C. Taylor:* A comparison of supratentorial intracranial meningiomas operated upon with and without induced hypothermia. Brit. J. Surgery *48* (1960), 155—157. — *McKissock, W., K. W. E. Paine,* and *L. S. Walsh:* The value of hypothermia in the surgical treatment of ruptured intracranial aneurysms. J. Neurosurg. *17* (1960), 700—707. — *Obrador, S., F. J. De Elio,* y *A. Garcia del Barrio:* Nuestra experienca con la hipotermia y la urea en la anestesia neuroquirurgica. Rev. Esp. de Oto-Neuro-Oftal. *124* (1962). — *Pool, J. L., J. Ransohoff, M. D. Yahr,* and *J. F. Hammill:* Early surgical treatment of aneurysms of the circle of Willis. Neurology *9* (1959), 478—486. — *Pool, J. L.:* Aneurysms of the anterior communicating artery. Bifrontal craniotomy and routine use of temporary clips. J. Neurosurg. *18* (1961), 98—111. — *Pool, J. L.:* Timing and techniques in the intracranial surgery of ruptured aneurysms of the anterior communicating artery. J. Neurosurg. *19* (1962), 378—388. — *Rosomoff, H. L.:* Protective effects of hypothermia against pathological processes of the nervous system. Ann. New York Acad. Sc. *80* (1959), 475—486. — *Rosomoff, H. L.,* and *J. Ransohoff:* Hypothermia in the surgery of third ventricle and parasellar area in children. Surg. Forum. *10* (1960), 748. — *Rosomoff, H. L.:* Effect of hypothermia and hypertonic urea on distribution of intracranial contents. J. Neurosurg. *18* (1961), 753—759. — *Rosomoff, H. L.:* Pathophysiology of the central nervous system during hypothermia. Acta Neurochirurgica, Suppl. XIII. Hypothermia in Neurosurgery. Wien: Springer. 1964. — *Sedzimir, C. F.,* and *J. W. Dundee:* Hypothermia in the treatment of cerebral tumors. J. Neurosurg. *15* (1958), 199—206. — *Uihlein, A., H. R. Terry,* and *J. T. Martin:* Induced hypothermia in neurologic conditions. Med. Clin. North Am. *44* (1960), 1079—1100. — *Vandewater, S. L., W. M. Lougheed, J. W. Scott,* and *E. H. Botterell:* Some observations with the use of hypothermia in neurosurgery. Anaes. and Analg. Curr. Res. *37* (1958), 29—36.

Ullevål Sykehus — Oslo (Norge)

Physiopathology, Methods and Clinical Results of Selective Brain Cooling

By

K. Kristiansen

With 8 Figures

General hypothermia in animals and man has been intensively investigated during the past ten years. The effects include lowering of the metabolic rate, slowing of the heart and respiration, decreased nervous conductivity and modifications of the electrolyte balance. Thus considerable changes of the "milieu interne" are taking place. The homeostatic derangement increases with decreasing temperatures and the biological limit to general hypothermia without the aid of extracorporeal circulation lies between 26—28° C. If lower temperatures are desirable without a cardio-pulmonary by-pass, local cooling of separate organs may be the method of choice. The cooling is thereby confined to the structures for which the hypothermia is essential, the low temperatures may be obtained rapidly and a precise control of the temperature level is possible.

The local cooling of separate organs may be said to originate from the old experience pertaining to local freezing of extremities to obtain anaesthesia in amputations. Cold injuries and peripheral vascular diseases with threatening gangrene have also been treated by local cooling of the affected parts to reduce the oxygen requirements of the damaged tissue.

Experimental selective cooling of internal organs has been accomplished by several authors with regard to the kidney, the heart and the brain. For the kidney reference may be made to publications by *Birkeland* et al. (1959), *Semb* (1959), *Semb jr.* et al. (1960), *Mitchell* and *Woodruff* (1957) and *Cockett* (1961). A special technique for local cooling of the kidney has also been applied by

Semb (1959) in patients with a single remaining kidney in whom clamping of the renal pedicle was required for a considerable length of time for the purpose of resection. The renal oxygen consumption is reduced approximately in an exponential way with the reduction of temperature.

The selective cooling of the heart through a cannula via the carotid or subclavian artery down to the origin of the coronary arteries has also resulted in a rapid reduction in oxygen consumption of the heart muscle (*Semb jr.*, 1961).

The many variables in the regulation of the cerebral blood flow, of the distal vascular pressure in the brain and of the oxygen consumption and metabolism of the brain make studies of the effects on this organ of selective hypothermia extremely complicated. Much of the knowledge gained in experimental and clinical work on general hypothermia may be applied for the physiological changes resulting from local cooling of the brain, but there are significant differences particularly with regard to the degree of cardio-vascular and metabolic reactions. From the extensive literature dealing with the effects on the brain of general cooling of the whole organism only a few pertinent data will be mentioned.

Rosomoff and *Holaday* (1954) noted a 75 per cent decrease in cerebral blood flow at rectal temperatures of about 26° C in surface-cooled dogs. They found very little change in the arterio-venous oxygen differences during this hypothermia, and came to the conclusion that hypothermia produced no hypoxia of brain tissue if adequate respiratory and cardiac functions were maintained. Another important observation by *Rosomoff* (1956) was an increase in the cerebral vascular resistance in dogs subjected to general cooling to 25° C. The same effect was found during cooling in monkeys (*Bering* et al., 1956).

Marshall, Owens and *Swan* (1956) tested the toleration to total arrest of blood flow to the brain for different periods in normothermic and hypothermic dogs, and concluded that hypothermia of 23—26° C produced a threefold increase in occlusion time based on survival and comparable brain changes when the arterial supply alone was occluded, and a twofold increase with simultaneous occlusion of the arterial and venous circulation. *Sweet, Brewster, Osgood* and *White* (1957) stressed the importance of slow cooling and re-warming. The effects on the electroencephalogram of lowered body temperature have also been amply studied (*Scott, McQueen* and *Callaghan*, 1953; *Ferrari* and *Amantea*, 1955).

Selective Brain Cooling in Animals

Several methods have been developed for localized cooling of the brain with the purpose of obtaining cerebral temperature levels which would represent a considerable risk under general hypothermia due to the high incidence of cardiac complications. The hazards of the methods of local cooling by perfusion are mainly due to cannulation of major vessels with the circulation of blood through an extracorporeal circuit and the necessary heparinization of the blood. *Woodhall* et al. (1958) achieved the selective cooling by a localized extracorporeal brain circulation with the carotid artery as afferent channel and the jugular vein as efferent channel. This method requires a separate oxygenator for the jugular blood which is re-circulated through the brain. A high morbidity and mortality rate was observed because of progressive hemolysis, the hazard of air embolism and the difficulty in maintaining a constant blood flow through the brain. A rapid fall in oxygen consumption was noted in the perfused brain, and at 20—21° C the arteriovenous oxygen differences were virtually zero. The cortex became electrically silent below 20—21° C.

Lourie et al. (1960) compared the surface brain temperatures with those in the interior of the cerebrum and the cerebellum, and tried to determine which physiological responses could be attributed to the selective brain cooling alone as compared with the total body cooling. These authors stressed the variable and prominent anastomoses between extra- and intracranial circulation in the dog. They abandoned the carotid-jugular perfusion method of *Woodhall* et al. in favor of the simpler carotid-carotid shunt. The average temperature difference between the two hemispheres in their experiments was 3.1° C and the temperature of the cerebellum also followed closely the level of the perfused cerebral hemisphere. The cooling of the perfused side proceeded at 0.47° C per minute which is considerably slower than the values found in our own experiments at Ullevål Hospital (*Lund* et al., 1958).

Geiger (1958) stressed the important metabolic contribution of other organs, especially the liver, to normal brain function, and warned against a too strictly isolated brain circulation.

Both for experimental and later for clinical purposes selective hypothermia of the brain has most frequently been accomplished by an arterio-arterial shunt. *Parkins, Jenssen* and *Vars* (1954) used a carotid-carotid shunt and circulated the blood through an extracorporeal cooling system to produce differential hypothermia. This method of cooling was well tolerated by the dogs and increased

the central nervous system resistance against anoxia. *Adams* and
Pevehouse (1959) induced regional hypothermia of the brain in
dogs and monkeys by the same method, and recorded intravascular
pressures, electrocardiogram, electroencephalogram and temperatures in the brain, in the rectum and in the muscle mass of the
right and left ventricles of the heart. Important parameters like
the rate of blood flow through the extracorporeal cooling circuit
and the perfusion pressure were not measured in these experiments.

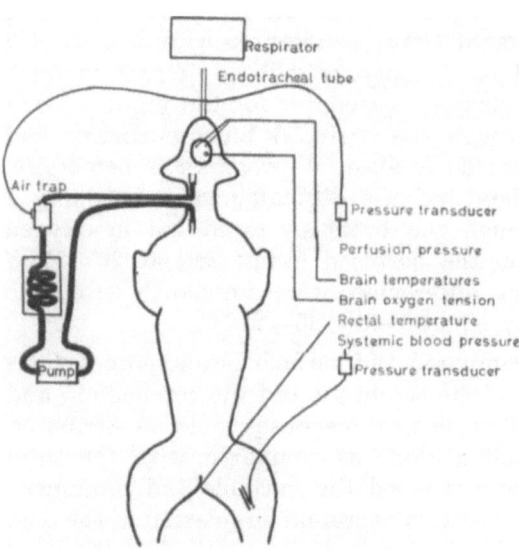

Fig. 1. Experimental arrangement for perfusing
the brain with cold and warm blood. (By courtesy
of *Lund, Johansen, Krog* and *Birkeland*, 1958)

Their conclusion was
that low temperatures
per se were not del-
eterious to the brain.

At Ulleval Hospi-
tal, Oslo, a series of
experiments with iso-
lated cooling of the
brain were carried out
in dogs from 1956
(*Lund, Johansen, Krog*
and *Birkeland*, 1958).
Polyethylene cathe-
ters were inserted into
the common carotid
artery, one in the
direction of the heart
and the other in the
direction of the brain,
and the catheters were
connected to an ex-
tracorporeal circuit
including a pump, a cooling coil and a bubble-trap (Fig. 1).

Different perfusion rates were obtained by adjusting the speed
of the pump according to a pre-calibrated scale. Perfusion pressure
and arterial blood pressure were registered continuously by means
of strain gauge manometers connected to the cranial end of the
extracorporeal circuit and to the femoral artery respectively.
Perfusion resistance was calculated from the perfusion pressure and
the volume flow, and stated in $\frac{\text{mm. Hg pressure}}{\text{ml. flow per minute}}$ = P.R.U. The
temperature was recorded from the brain, the perfusing blood and
the rectum.

During the cooling procedure an initial increase in the vascular
resistance of the brain was observed (Fig. 2).

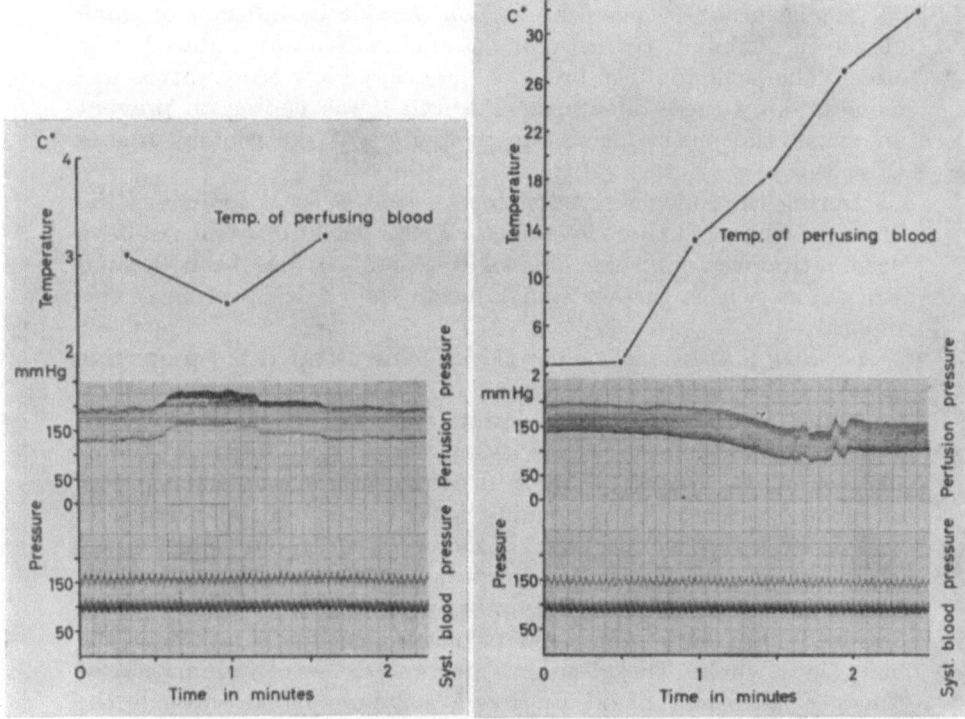

Fig. 2. Response of perfusion pressure to cold and to warm blood.
(By courtesy of *Lund, Johansen, Krog* and *Birkeland*, 1958)

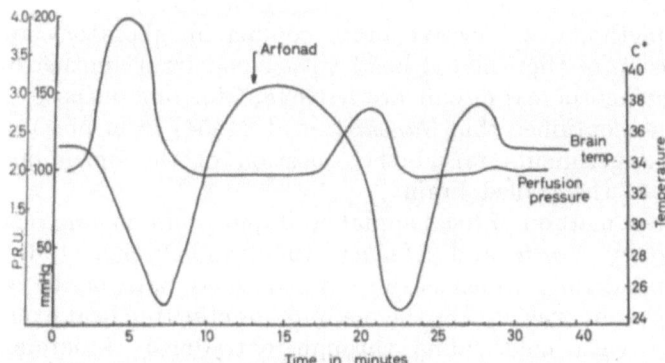

Fig. 3. Temperature of the brain and perfusion pressure in a dog perfused
through one common carotid artery with a volume flow of 7 ml. per kilogram
per minute. The first cooling and warming carried out without Arfonad and
the second cooling and warming while 5 drops per minute of Arfonad 50 mg.
per 100 ml. saline were administered intravenously. (By courtesy of *Lund,
Johansen, Krog* and *Birkeland*, 1958)

144   K. Kristiansen:

Inhalation of 10 per cent carbon dioxide or infusion of small doses of Arfonad (trimetaphancamphorsulfonate) reduced this effect. The cooling of the brain to the desired low temperature was facilitated by these agents, and Arfonad was chosen to prevent anoxia of the brain during the first stage of the cooling process (Fig. 3).

During the following years this method of local cooling of the brain has been further developed. Technical improvements have been introduced and the clinical applicability has been demonstrated, as will be further elucidated in the clinical section of this report.

Connolly, Boyd and *Calvin* (1962) demonstrated the protective effect of low brain temperatures in dogs during total cerebral ischemia. Six animals whose brains were cooled to 10° C by an extracorporeal femoral-carotid shunt, survived 60 minutes of complete circulatory arrest. *White* and *Donald* (1962) studied the effect of isolated cerebral hypothermia on the cardiovascular system. It was possible to cool the brain preferentially without reducing the body temperature to levels at which cardiac irregularity became a serious consideration, and deep brain temperatures of 15° C were obtained with only minor reductions in the temperature of the body as a whole. These authors prevented the contamination of the cold perfusing blood by warm systemic blood through the application of clamps on the brachiocephalic and the left subclavian arteries, and ligation of the first four or five pairs of intercostal arteries and both internal mammary arteries according to the method of *Marshall, Owens* and *Swan* (1956).

The methods of selective brain cooling in laboratory animals by perfusion of the isolated head with blood from another animal in the extracorporeal circuit are irrelevant for our purpose. But it should be mentioned that *Gänshirt* et al. (1954) from observations in such experiments raised the question of the optimum temperature of the cooled brain.

Another method of local spinal cord and brain cooling has been suggested by *Negrin* and *Klauber* (1960) and *Negrin* (1961). The cerebrospinal fluid which is the natural water bath of the central nervous system was used as the medium for effecting heat exchange. Perfusion with cold saline through extradural catheters gave effective protection against ischaemia of the spinal cord. The cerebral hemispheres were cooled in a similar fashion by circulating the cold solution through catheters placed in the subdural and ventricular spaces. With a different purpose *Tokuoka, Aoki, Higashi* and *Tatebayashi* (1961) irrigated the cerebral ventricular system and investigated the unresponsiveness caused by the cooling.

Ommaya and *Baldwin* (1963) have used a direct extravascular local brain cooling by constant irrigation in cats, rabbits, monkeys and man, and have been able to demonstrate the protective effect of such hypothermia against ischaemia. According to their opinion extravascular brain cooling is physiologically a more justifiable technique than the intravascular cooling and it has the advantage that it can be applied when required instead of throughout a long-lasting operation.

Clinical Application of Selective Brain Cooling

The *clinical* use of local cooling of brain tissue was introduced in the late thirties by *Temple Fay* who gave a vivid report of his early experiences at a meeting of the *Harvey Cushing Society* in 1958 (*Fay*, 1959). This localized refrigeration was applied in patients with intracranial infections and tumors.

In spite of the fairly extensive experimental experience in laboratory animals the reports on application of selective cooling to the human brain are still few. *Kimoto, Sugie* and *Asano* (1956) were encouraged by their results in experimental work to operate on patients with congenital heart disease with the aid of selective brain cooling. According to *Connolly, Boyd* and *Calvin* (1962) *Kimoto* has subsequently employed this method in more than 70 patients subjected to open-heart surgery. From the discussion following the paper by *Connolly* et al. it appears that *Adams* and *Wylie* have used regional cerebral hypothermia in five intracranial operations. In the four human cases reported by *Connolly* et al. (1962) the carotid and vertebral arteries were isolated in the neck and separately clamped according to the requirements during the intracranial procedure. *Adams* and *Wylie* (1959) prefer a technique in which the innominate artery and the left carotid and subclavian arteries are clamped beneath the manubrium of the sternum and they recommend total arterial inflow occlusion prior to attacking the intracranial lesion rather than waiting for hemorrhage to occur.

Personal Material

The main reason for local brain cooling in humans is the possibility that temporary arrest of the blood circulation through one of the major arteries may be required during the operation. The period of controlled hypotension may also be prolonged beyond that which can be safely permitted when the temperature is normal.

Our laboratory experiences with selective brain cooling in dogs seemed to warrant the application of the method in patients. Even with brain temperatures down to 11° C the animals showed no signs of brain damage. In 1958 we decided to use this technique in patients with the following indications:

1) Large and deep-seated arteriovenous aneurysms.

2) Selected cases of saccular aneurysms on the internal carotid artery or its branches.

3) Highly vascularized tumors infiltrating the major vessels at the base of the brain.

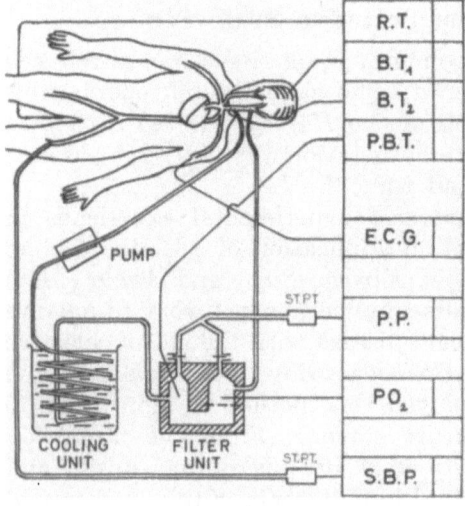

Fig. 4. Diagram of selective cooling of the brain by perfusion

The perfusion technique in man is essentially the same as in the experimental animals. Blood from the common carotid artery is diverted along a cannula by means of a roller pump through the cooling coil, the filter and a bubble trap and thence to the internal carotid artery via a second cannula (Fig. 4).

The perfusion unit has been gradually developed from a simple manually controlled pump and improvisation for each case to be operated upon. When the cooling procedure had been established as a routine method the need for a special set-up for selective cooling of the brain became necessary. The filter unit has previously been described by *Krog* and *Kristiansen* (1962) and the final model of the servo-operated perfusion unit has recently been described by *Krog* et al. (1962). During long operations the adjustment of the perfusion pressure and the cerebral blood flow is secured by electronic means to prevent an undesirable rise in the perfusion pressure (Fig. 5).

In addition to the arterial pressure and the perfusion pressure readings and the continuous temperature recordings, samples may be taken from both the systemic arterial blood and from the blood in the extracorporeal circuit for measurement of arterial oxygen saturation, pH, pCO_2, fibrinolysis, platelet counts etc. The apparatus is primed with 300 ml. heparinized blood, and shortly before starting the extracorporeal circulation heparin is given intravenously. If required, Arfonad may be given as a slow intravenous drip of a solution containing 0.5 mg. per ml. When Fluothane is used as an anesthetic Arfonad may be dispensed with because the initial reaction of the brain vessels to the introduction of cold blood into the carotid system is negligible.

The perfusion rate in our patients has varied from 150 to 200 ml. blood per minute. During the selective cooling through one carotid artery it is an advantage to perfuse the side of the brain to be

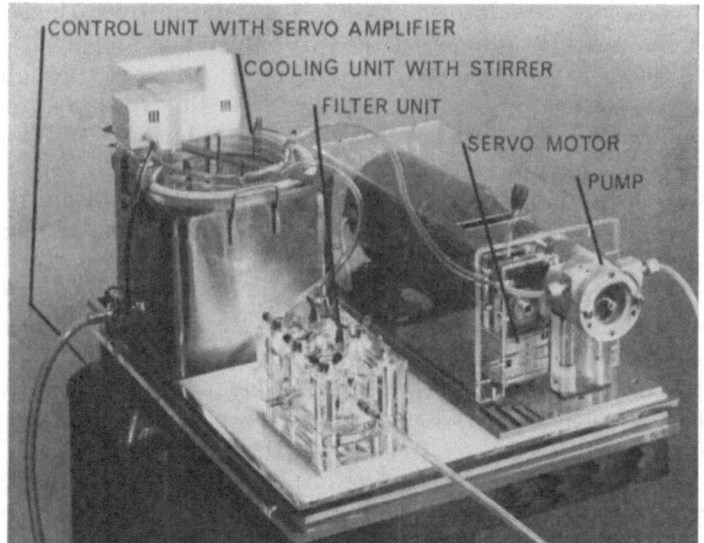

Fig. 5. Servo-operated perfusion unit

cooled with a somewhat higher pressure than the systemic blood pressure. In this way the blood is prevented from being forced from other parts of the brain to the side of perfusion and thus counteract effective cooling. Recently low molecular dextran, 50 ml. per kilogram, has been given during the operation to prevent the possible tendency of aggregation and sludging of the red blood cells (Løfstrøm, 1959).

Satisfactory cooling of the perfused hemisphere has been obtained usually within 10—15 minutes. The temperature has been kept at about 20° C, sometimes a little above, sometimes lower down to 17° C. In two patients in whom a bilateral frontal exposure was necessary it was possible to measure the temperature also in

the contralateral hemisphere. The temperature of the other half
of the brain followed the cooled side with a few degrees centigrade
difference, but a differential cooling may occur (Fig. 8). Comparison
between the temperature of the white substance and the temperature
on the surface of the cortex has been performed. The temperature
in the interior of the brain in these cases was constantly a little
lower than the brain surface temperature, perhaps owing to a
certain heating effect by conduction from the scalp and the skull
which are supplied by blood of normal temperature via collaterals
from the external carotid artery of the other side.

No attempts have been made to perform parts of the operations
during complete circulatory arrest. Most of the operations were
carried out with little hemorrhage on a shrunken and firm brain.

In 9 cases a temporary arrest of the blood flow through the
perfused side has been necessary due to bleeding from a ruptured
artery. In one case also the contralateral carotid artery was exposed
to allow temporary clamping of the blood flow on both sides. If
bleeding occurs a bloodless field has thus not been obtained, but
it has been relatively easy to control the hemorrhage because of
the low blood pressure induced in the ruptured vessel when the
extracorporeal circulation is interrupted. It is also possible to clamp
temporarily the artery supplying the field of operation when the
proximal part of the artery is exposed.

Since 1958 we have operated upon 27 patients under selective
hypothermia. The material consists of 16 patients with saccular
aneurysms of different locations, 8 arteriovenous malformations
and 3 malignant gliomas. Selection of patients for local cooling has
been done according to the possible risk of uncontrollable hemorrhage during the operative intervention. These narrow indications
are reflected in the fact that no patient with meningioma has been
subjected to local cooling. The three patients with malignant
gliomas all died a few days after the operation because of the
extensive tumor infiltration of neighbouring areas of the brain.
All the patients with arteriovenous malformations have recovered.
Such malformations seem to represent the most suitable cases for
selective brain cooling because they attract so much of the perfusing blood that the cooling is very rapidly established.

Of the 16 patients operated upon for saccular aneurysms 3 must
be regarded as operative fatalities.

The hazards of the method are mainly connected with the
cannulation of the carotid artery. One patient developed a thrombosis of the internal carotid artery caused by intimal damage from
a too large catheter tip. She died from infarction of the left hemi-

sphere a few days after the operation in spite of the pre-operative demonstration of a good collateral circulation from the arteries on the other side. To prevent intimal damage it is important to use catheters which permit an easy insertion and passage through the lumen of the internal carotid artery.

Two post-operative deaths were due to a diffuse intracranial hemorrhage. This complication which is well known in extra-corporeal circulation and which is also a potential danger in hypothermia, is of particular significance in neurosurgical operations. The actual cause of the bleeding in these cases was uncertain. Thrombocyte counts were normal and no increased fibrinolytic

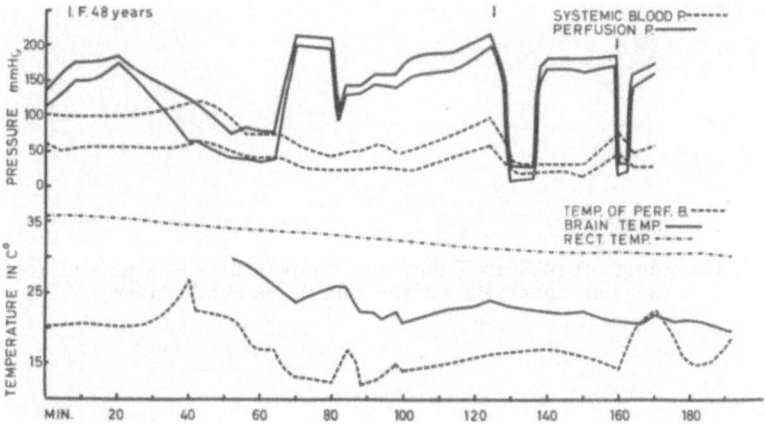

Fig. 6. Tracings of temperature and pressure during operation in a patient with a large arteriovenous malformation. Temporary interruption of perfusion at 130 minutes and at 160 minutes

activity was present. The remaining heparin had been carefully titrated and neutralized at the end of the procedure. A careful re-testing of the neutralizing effect of protamine sulphate or polybren is always necessary.

Figs. 6, 7 and 8 show representative recordings during selective brain hypothermia in three patients. One patient (Fig. 6) had a large arteriovenous malformation in the left frontal lobe including the motor speech area. Because of profuse bleeding from a ruptured artery the perfusion was stopped, first during a ten minutes period and then during a five minutes period to control the hemorrhage and ligate the bleeding vessel.

Fig. 7 shows the smooth course of the cooling in a patient with a large saccular aneurysm on the right middle cerebral artery.

In this case the dissection of the aneurysm was fraught with danger
due to the intimate relationship of the two main branches of the
artery with the entire aneurysmal wall.

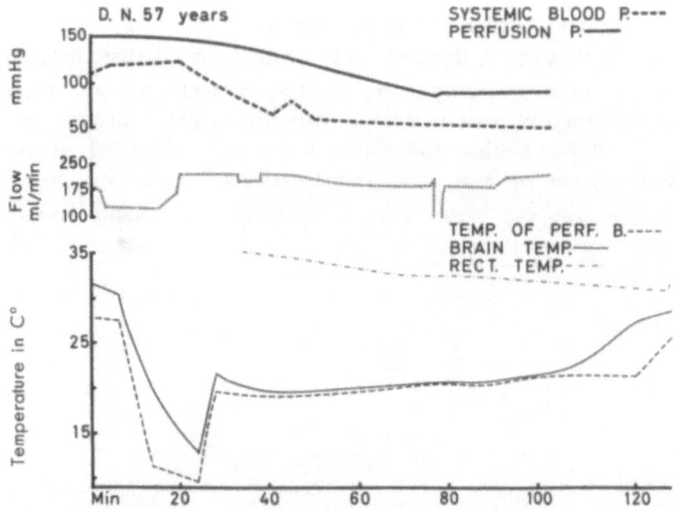

Fig. 7. Recordings of pressures, flow and temperatures in a patient with a
saccular aneurysm on the middle cerebral artery

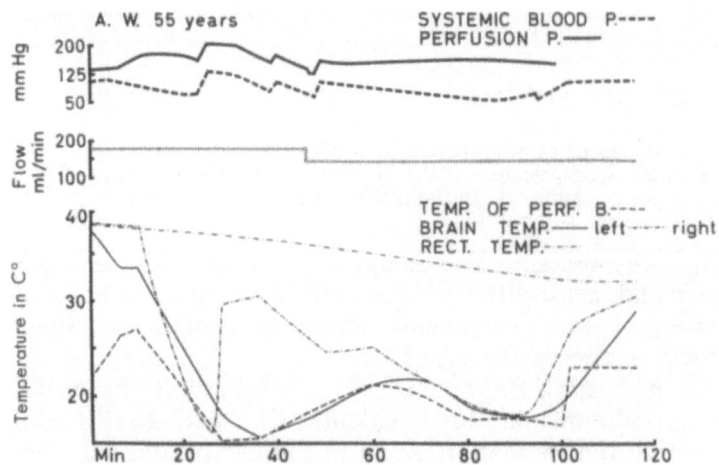

Fig. 8. Temperature recordings in both halves of the brain in a patient with
a frontal glioblastoma

In Fig. 8 are presented recordings from a patient with a bilateral
frontal glioma in whom it was possible to register the temperature
also from the contralateral hemisphere. The separation of the two

temperature curves during the second half hour of the perfusion indicates an obstruction to the blood flow through the circle of Willis, perhaps due to simultaneous operative manipulations in this region.

More detailed information about some of our patients has been published previously (*Kristiansen, Krog* and *Lund,* 1960; *Kristiansen,* 1961; and *Lund* and *Kristiansen,* 1962). This method of local brain cooling seems to be relatively safe and practicable but requires a team experienced in extracorporeal cooling technique. On the other hand, if bleeding occurs during the operation, it is as a rule not possible with our procedure to obtain a completely dry field such as may be achieved if total circulatory arrest is secured by preliminary clamping of the four large arteries in the neck. Even in these cases however some blood may reach the cranium through vertebral anastomotic channels.

The cannulation of the carotid arteries carries some risks. In the future we may change to a femoral-carotid shunt with the afferent catheter in one femoral artery and the afferent catheter inserted through the external carotid into the common carotid artery, which then will be clamped proximal to the catheter tip.

No complications have occurred from the side of the heart, not even temporary arrhythmias. The systemic blood pressure has been readily maintained at levels which must be regarded as physiological at the actual level of the brain temperature. The local cerebral hypothermia and the long perfusion time in many patients had no significant influence upon the morphology or on the registered biochemical properties of the blood.

Summary

Selective cooling of particular internal organs as an alternative to general hypothermia during operative interventions confines the hypothermia to the structures for which the lowered temperature is essential. Cardiac complications and metabolic disturbances which are apt to occur in general hypothermia below 28° C may thus be avoided. Cannulation of major vessels, circulation of blood through an extracorporeal circuit and heparinization must on the other hand be considered as possible hazards of the methods of local cooling by perfusion.

Selective cooling of the brain with normal or only moderately lowered temperature of the rest of the body has been performed experimentally in animals in several laboratories. Through local cooling temperature levels of the brain may readily be obtained which would represent a considerable risk under general hypothermia. Cerebral hypothermia has been induced with different methods. A localized extracorporeal brain circulation with the carotid artery as afferent channel and the jugular vein as efferent channel requires a separate oxygenator for the jugular blood which is recirculated through the brain. This method carries a high morbidity and mortality rate due to progressive hemolysis, the hazard of air embolism and difficulty in maintaining a constant blood flow through the brain.

The cooling irrigation of the brain stems from *Temple Fay*'s pioneer observations before the second world war. The procedures include irrigation of the ventricular system and the subdural space, and the direct extravascular regional cortical cooling. These methods have been applied successfully in clinical neurosurgery in a few cases.

Both for experimental and clinical purposes selective hypothermia of the brain has most frequently been accomplished by an arterio-arterial shunt. By way of a catheter inserted into the common carotid artery or into the femoral artery blood is removed and circulated through an extracorporeal cooling system. Through another catheter which is guided from the common carotid into the internal carotid artery the cold blood is then conducted to the brain.

The protective effect of the selective hypothermia in preventing ischemic brain damage, has been well established. Several reports have been published describing more or less complete temporary arrest of the blood flow to the brain for periods which in normothermic brains would have resulted in fatal ischemic changes.

At Ullevål Hospital in Oslo selective brain cooling has been accomplished in 27 patients through an extracorporeal carotid-carotid shunt. Indications for local hypothermia were considered to be present in patients with large and deep-seated arterio-venous malformations, in selected cases of saccular aneurysms and in patients with richly vascularized tumors infiltrating around the major intracranial vessels. The temperature of the brain has been lowered to 20 degrees or below while the general body temperature has been only moderately affected, even during perfusions lasting for three hours or more. No complications have been observed due to the free return of the cooled blood to the right side of the heart. Continuous registrations of brain and body temperatures, of systemic blood pressure and perfusion pressure, pulse rate, electrocardiogram and in some cases electroencephalogram have been made. Data have been obtained from blood analysis with regard to arterial oxygen saturation, pH, pCO_2, standard bicarbonate, thrombocyte counts and fibrinolytic activity. The perfusion unit and the cooling procedure, the beneficial effects and the complications of the method are described and discussed in relation to other techniques of inducing selective cerebral hypothermia.

Zusammenfassung

Die selektive Unterkühlung einzelner innerer Organe als Alternative zur allgemeinen Hypothermie während operativer Eingriffe beschränkt die Hypothermie auf diejenigen Strukturen, für die eine Temperatursenkung wesentlich ist. Auf diese Weise werden kardiale Komplikationen und Stoffwechselstörungen, die als Folge einer allgemeinen Hypothermie unter 28° C auftreten können, vermieden. Die Kanülierung großer Gefäße, die Zirkulation des Blutes durch einen extrakorporalen Kreislauf und die Heparinisierung müssen anderseits als mögliche Risiken der örtlichen Perfusionsunterkühlung in Betracht gezogen werden.

Selektive Unterkühlung des Gehirns bei normaler oder nur wenig gesenkter Temperatur des übrigen Körpers wurde in mehreren Laboratorien tierexperimentell ausgeführt. Es lassen sich mit dieser Methode im Gehirn Temperaturgrade erreichen, die mittels allgemeiner Hypothermie nur unter erheblichem Risiko verwirklicht werden können.

Zerebrale Hypothermie ist auf verschiedene Weise durchgeführt worden. Eine selektive extrakorporale Hirnzirkulation mit der Arteria carotis als afferentem und der Vena jugularis als efferentem Schenkel erfordert einen eigenen Oxygenator für das Jugularisblut, das dann wieder durch das Hirn zirkuliert. Diese Methode ist mit einer hohen Morbidität und Mortalität belastet, bedingt durch fortschreitende Hämolyse, das Risiko von Luftembolie und die Schwierigkeit, eine konstante Durchströmung des Gehirnes aufrechtzuerhalten.

Die Methode der Spülungsunterkühlung des Hirnes entstammt den bahnbrechenden Untersuchungen von *Temple Fay* aus der Zeit vor dem zweiten Weltkrieg. Das Verfahren beinhaltet die Durchspülung des Ventrikelsystems und des Subduralraumes mit kalter Flüssigkeit und die umschriebene extravaskuläre Kühlung der Hirnrinde. Sie ist in einigen wenigen Fällen erfolgreich in der klinischen Neurochirurgie angewendet worden.

Sowohl für experimentelle wie auch für klinische Zwecke ist die selektive Hirnunterkühlung am häufigsten mittels eines arterio-arteriellen Shunts ausgeführt worden. Über einen Katheter, der in die Arteria carotis communis oder die Arteria femoralis eingeführt ist, wird Blut in ein extrakorporales Kühlungssystem geleitet. Durch einen weiteren Katheter, der von der Arteria carotis communis aus in die Arteria carotis interna vorgeschoben wird, gelangt das kalte Blut dann zum Gehirn.

Der Schutzeffekt der selektiven Hirnkühlung gegen das Auftreten ischiämischer Hirnschäden hat sich gut bestätigt. Es wurden mehrere Berichte veröffentlicht, die eine mehr oder weniger vollständige vorübergehende Unterbrechung der zerebralen Zirkulation für Zeitspannen beschreiben, die bei einem Gehirn normaler Temperatur zu tödlichen ischiämischen Veränderungen geführt haben würden.

Im Ulleval Hospital in Oslo ist die selektive Hirnunterkühlung bei 27 Patienten mit Hilfe eines extrakorporalen Shunts von und zur Karotis durchgeführt worden.

Als Indikation zur selektiven Hypothermie galten sehr große und tiefliegende arterio-venöse Gefäßmißbildungen, manche Fälle mit sackförmigen

Aneurysmen und Fälle mit stark vaskularisierten Tumoren, welche die
großen intrakraniellen Gefäße umwachsen hatten. Die Hirntemperatur
wurde auf 20° C oder tiefer gesenkt, während die allgemeine Körpertemperatur nur wenig beeinflußt wurde, selbst wenn die Perfusion 3 Stunden oder
länger andauerte. Es wurden keine Komplikationen gesehen, die auf das
freie Rückfließen des gekühlten Blutes zum rechten Herzen zurückzuführen
wären. Fortlaufend wurden Hirn- und Körpertemperatur, allgemeiner Blut-
druck und Perfusionsdruck, Pulsfrequenz, EKG und in manchen Fällen auch
EEG registriert. Außerdem wurden arterielle Sauerstoffsättigung, Blut-pH,
pCO_2, Standart Bicarbonat, Thrombozytenzahl und fibrinolytische Aktivität wiederholt bestimmt. Das Perfusionsgerät und der Kühlungsvorgang,
die positiven Wirkungen und die Komplikationen der Methode wurden be-
schrieben und im Vergleich mit anderen Verfahren der selektiven zerebralen
Hypothermie diskutiert.

Résumé

Le refroidissement sélectif d'organes internes particuliers en tant que
substitution de l'hypothermie générale durant des interventions limite
l'hypothermie aux structures pour lesquelles la température abaissée est
essentielle. Les complications cardiaques et les troubles métaboliques qui
peuvent apparaitre dans l'hypothermie générale au-dessous de 28° C, peuvent
ainsi être évités. La canulation des vaisseaux majeurs, la circulation du sang
par un circuit extra corporel et l'héparinisation doivent d'autre part, être
considérées comme des risques possibles des méthodes de refroidissement
local par perfusion.

Le refroidissement sélectif du cerveau avec une température normale
ou seulement peu abaissée du reste du corps a été réalisé expérimentalement
sur des animaux dans plusieurs laboratoires. Par le refroidissement local,
on peut facilement obtenir des niveaux de température du cerveau qui
présenteraient un risque considérable sous hypothermie générale. L'hypothermie cérébrale a été produite avec différentes méthodes. Une circulation
cérébrale extracorporelle localisée avec l'artère carotide comme canal afférent
et la veine jugulaire comme canal efférent demande un oxygénateur séparé
pour le sang jugulaire qui est remis en circulation dans le cerveau. Cette
méthode comporte un taux élevé de morbidité et de mortalité dû à l'hyme-
lyse progressive, le risque d'une embolie (par air) et de la difficulté à main-
tenir une circulation constante du sang à travers le cerveau.

L'irrigation pour refroidir le cerveau remonte aux observations du pion-
nier Temple Fay avant la seconde guerre mondiale. Les façons de procédés
comprennent l'irrigation du système ventriculaire et de l'espace subdural,
et le refroidissement directement extravasculaire de la région corticale.

Ces méthodes ont été appliquées avec succès dans quelques cas de neurochirurgie clinique.

Dans des buts à la fois expérimentaux et cliniques l'hypothermie sélective
du cerveau a été la plus fréquemment réalisée par un circuit (un shunt)
artério-artériel. Au moyen d'un "catheter" inséré dans l'artère carotide ou
dans l'artère fémorale, le sang est dévié et mis en circulation à travers un
système de refroidissement extracorporel. A travers un autre catheter qui
est guidé de la simple artère carotide dans l'artère carotide interne, le sang
froid est alors conduit au cerveau.

L'effet protecteur de l'hypothermie sélective qu'empêche les troubles
chimiques du cerveau a bien été établi. Plusieurs rapports ont été publiés
décrivant des arrêts temporaires plus ou moins complets de l'écoulement

sanguin dans le cerveau pendant des périodes qui dans des cerveaux normothermiques auraient entrainé des changements chimiques fatals.

A l'Hôpital d'Ulleval à Oslo, on a réalisé le refroidissement sélectif du cerveau sur 27 malades par un shunt extracorporel carotide à carotide.

On a considéré des indications pour l'hypothermie locale qui se présentaient chez des malades avec de larges et profondes malformations artério-veineuses, dans des cas choisis d'anévrisme sacculaire et chez des malades ayant des tumeurs frotement vascularisées s'infiltrant vers les vaisseaux majeurs intercraniens. La température du cerveau a été abaissée de 20° et plus tandis que la température générale du corps a été seulement modérément affectée même durant des perfusions de 3 heures ou plus. Aucune complication n'a été observée dûe au libre retour du sang refroidi au côté droit du cœur. Des contrôles continuels de la température du corps et du cerveau, de la pression sanguine et de la pression de la perfusion, de la vitesse du pouls, un électrocardiogramme et dans certains cas un électro-encéphalogramme ont été faits.

On a obtenu des données d'après l'analyse du sang quant à la saturation artérielle d'oxygène, Ph, PCO^2, bicarbonate standard, calculs des thrombocytes et activité fibrinolytique. L'unité de perfusion et le procédé de refroidissement, les effets bénéfiques et les complications de la méthode sont décrits et discutés avec d'autres techniques d'hypothermie cérébrale sélective.

Riassunto

Il raffreddamento selettivo di particolari organi interni, anzichè l'ipotermia generale, durante interventi chirurgici, limita l'ipotermia a quelle strutture per le quali è essenziale un abbassamento della temperatura. Possono così essere evitate le complicanze cardiache e metaboliche, che d, solito si verificano in ipotermia generalizzata al di sotto di 28° C. D'altra parte l'incannulamento di grossi vasi, la circolazione del sangue attraverso un circuito extracorporeo e l'eparinizzazione devono essere considerati come possibile cause di complicazioni del metodo di raffreddamento locale mediante perfusione.

Il raffreddamento selettivo del cervello con temperatura normale oi solo di poco abbassata nel resto del corpo, è stato ottenuto sperimentalmente in diversi laboratori. Con questo metodo si possono ottenere dei livelli di raffreddamento nel cervello, che sarebbero ottenuti solo con rischi gravissimi in condizioni di ipotermia generalizzata.

L'ipotermia cerebrale è stata ottenuta con diversi metodi. Una circolazione extracorporea cerebrale con la carotide, come canale afferente, e la giugulare, come efferente, richiede un ossigenatore indipendente per il sangue proveniente dalla giugulare, che viene di nuovo fatto ricircolare nell'encefalo. Questo metodo ha però un'alta mortalità per la progressiva emolisi, il pericolo di embolie e la difficoltà di mantenere un flusso ematico costante nell'encefalo.

Il raffreddamento per irrigazione deriva dalle osservazioni pionieristiche di *Temple Fay* eseguite prima della seconda guerra mondiale. Questo metodo comprende l'irrigazione del sistema ventricolare e degli spazi subdurali ed il raffreddamento extravascolare regionale corticale. Esso è stato usato con successo in neurochirurgia clinica in pochi casi.

Sia per scopi clinici che per scopi sperimentali l'ipotermia selettiva del cervello deve essere ottenuta mediante uno shunt arterio-arterioso. Il sangue viene prelevato mediante un catetere inserito nella carotide comune o nella femorale e fatto circolare attraverso un circuito raffreddante esterno. Attraverso un altro catetere, che viene spinto dalla carotide comune nella carotide interna, il sangue raffreddato viene fatto giungere al cervello.

L'effetto protettivo dell'ipotermia distrettuale nel prevenire un danno cerebrale ischemico è stato ben stabilito. Sono stati pubblicati molti lavori che descrivono l'arresto più o meno completo del flusso ematico cerebrale per periodi di tempo che avrebbero provocato danni ischemici fatali in cervelli normotermici.

All'Ospedale Ulleval di Oslo il raffreddamento cerebrale distrettuale è stato effettuato in 27 pazienti mediante uno shunt carotido-carotideo. Indicazioni per questo tipo di ipotermia sono stati le malformazioni artero-venose larghe e profonde, aneurismi sacculari e tumori molto vascolarizzati infiltranti, posti in vicinanza dei maggiori vasi intracranici. La temperatura del cervello è stata abbassata a 20 gradi, mentre la temperatura generale corporea è stata influenzata solo di poco, anche durante perfusioni durate tre ore o più. Nessuna complicazione si è avuta per il ritorno del sangue raffreddato nel cuore destro. Sono state fatte registrazioni continue della temperatura cerebrale e corporea, della pressione sistemica e della pressione di perfusione, della frequenza del polso, dell'elettrocardiogramma ed in qualche caso dell'elettroencefalogramma. Sono anche stati ottenuti dati riguardanti la tensione di ossigeno nel sangue arterioso, il Ph, il pCO_2, i bicarbonati e l'attività fibirnolitica. Vengono anche descritti l'apparecchio di perfusione ed il procedimento del raffreddamento, e vengono discussi i vantaggi e le complicazioni del metodo in rapporto ad altri metodi di ipotermia distrettuale cerebrale.

Resumen

El enfriamiento selectivo de determinados organos internos durante intervenciones quirúrgicas aparece como método alternante a la hipotermia general. Las complicaciones cardiacas y alteraciones metabólicas que pueden aparecer en la hipotermia general por debajo de 28° C pueden evitarse. Por otro lado la canulación de vasos importantes, la circulación de sangre por circuitos extracorporeos y la heparinización deben considerarse como posibles riesgos de los métodos del enfriamiento selectivo por perfusión.

El enfriamiento selectivo del cerebro con temperaturas normales o solamente con descenso moderado de la temperatura del resto del organismo se ha practicado en animales de laboratorio. Se han podido obtener descensos locales de la temperatura del cerebro que representarian un riesgo considerable con hipotermia general. La hipotermia cerebral ha sido obtenida por diferentes métodos. Una circulación extracorpórea localizada al cerebro con la arteria carótida como canal aferente y la vena yugular como canal eferente requiere un oxigenador separado para la sangre de la yugular cuando se recircula a través del cerebro. Este método acarrea un gran porcentaje de morbilidad y mortalidad por la progresiva hemolisis, el riesgo de embolias gaseosas y la dificultad para mantener un flujo constante de sangre al cerebro.

El enfriamiento del cerebro por irrigación data de las observaciones pioneras de TEMPLE FAY antes de la segunda guerra mundial. Los procedimientos incluyen la irrigación del sistema ventricular y del espacio subdural, así como el enfriamiento regional cortical extravascular directo. Estos métodos han sido aplicados con exito en unos pocos casos clínicos.

Tanto con métodos experimentales como clínicos la hipotermia selectiva del cerebro ha sido más frecuentemente realizada por un shunt arterio-arterial. Por medio de un catéter insertado en la arteria carótida común ó en la arteria femoral se extrae la sangre que se hace circular en un sistema de enframiento extracorpóreo. Por medio de otro catéter dirigido desde la arteria carótida común a la carótida interna la sangre fria se hace pasar al cerebro.

Los efectos protectores de la hipotermia selectiva para prevenir las lesiones isquémicas del cerebro ha sido bien establecido. Se han publicado varios trabajos describiendo paradas más o menos completas del flujo sanguineo al cerebro durante periodos en los cuales en cerebros normotérmicos se habian producido cambios isquémicos fatales.

En el Hospital Ulleval de Oslo el enfriamiento selectivo del cerebro se ha llevado a cabo en 27 enfermos por medio de un circuito extracorpóreo carótido-carótídeo. Las indicaciones para hipotermia local eran las malformaciones arterio-venosas grandes y profundas, algunos casos de aneurismas saculares y algunos tumores vascularizados e infiltrantes alrededor de grandes vasos intracraneales. La temperatura del cerebro llegaba a 20° o menos mientras la temperatura corpórea se afectaba muy discretamente, aún durante perfusiones que duraban tres horas o más. No se han visto complicaciones debidas al retorno de la sangre fria al corazón derecho. Se han hecho registros continuos de las temperaturas del cerebro y corpóreas, presión arterial y presión de perfusión, electrocardiograma y electroencefalograma en algunos casos. Se han obtenido datos en relación con la saturación de oxigeno arterial, pH, pCO_2, standard de bicarbonato, contajes de trombocitos y de actividad fibrinolítica. Se describen la unidad de perfusión y de enfriamiento junto con las complicaciones del método en relación a otras técnicas para producir hipotermia cerebral selectiva.

References

Adams, J. E., and *B. C. Pevehouse:* Regional hypothermia of the brain. Clinical Neurosurgery, Proc. Congr. Neurol. Surgeons, San Francisco, Calif. 1958. Chapter IV, pp. 104—118. Baltimore: The Williams & Wilkins Company. 1959. — *Adams, J.E.*, and *E. J. Wylie:* cit. *Connolly, Boyd* and *Calvin*, 1962. — *Bering, E. A., J. A. Taren, J. McMurrey*, and *W. F. Berhard:* The effect of hypothermia on the general physiology and cerebral metabolism of monkeys in the hypothermic state. Surg. Gyn. Obst. *102* (1956), 134— 138. — *Birkeland, S., A. Vogt, J. Krog*, and *C. Semb:* Renal circulatory occlusion and local cooling. J. Appl. Physiol. *14* (1959), 227—232. — *Cockett, A. T. K.:* The kidney and regional hypothermia. Surgery *50* (1961), 905— 910. — *Connolly, J. E., R. J. Boyd*, and *J. W. Calvin:* The protective effect of hypothermia in cerebral ischemia: Experimental and clinical application by selective brain cooling in the human. Surgery *52* (1962), 15—23. — *Fay, T.:* Early experiences with local and generalized refrigeration of the human brain. J. Neurosurg. *16* (1959), 239—259. — *Ferrari, E.*, and *L. Amantea:* Convulsive electrocortical discharges in hypothermic dog. Electroenceph. clin. Neurophysiol. 7 (1955), 441—448. — *Geiger, A.:* Correlation of brain metabolism and function by use of a brain perfusion method in situ. Physiol. Rev. *38* (1958), 1—20. — *Gänshirt, H., W. Krenkel, M. Schneider* und *W. Zylka:* Über den Einfluß der Temperatursenkung auf die Erholungsfähigkeit des Warmblütergehirns. Arch. exper. Path. u. Pharmakol. *222* (1954), 431— 449. — *Kimoto, S.:* cit. *Connolly, Boyd* and *Calvin*, 1962. — *Kimoto, S., S. Sugie*, and *K. Asano:* Open heart surgery under direct vision with the aid of brain-cooling by irrigation. Surgery *39* (1956), 592—603. — *Kristiansen, K.:*

Selective cooling of organs with special reference to the brain. J. Roy. Coll. Surg. of Edinburgh 7 (1961), 1—18. — *Kristiansen, K., J. Krog*, and *I. Lund:* Experiences with selective cooling of the brain. Acta chir. Scandinav. 1960, Suppl. 253, pp. 151—161. — *Krog, J.*, and *B. Kristiansen:* A new filter unit for extracorporeal circulation. J. Oslo City Hosp. *12* (1962), 108—111. — *Krog, J., S. Leraand, B. Kristiansen*, and *K. Kristiansen:* A servo-operated perfusion unit for selective cooling of the brain. J. Oslo City Hosp. *12* (1962), 238—243. — *Lourie, H., T. G. Holmes, W. Weinstein, H. G. Schwartz*, and *J. L. O'Leary:* Observations on selective brain cooling in dogs. A. M. A. Arch. Neurol. *3* (1960), 163—176. — *Lund, I., K. Johansen, J. Krog*, and *S. Birkeland:* The change in vascular resistance of the dog's brain on perfusion with cold blood and the modifying effect of CO_2 and trimetaphancamphorsulphonate (Arfonad®). Acta anaesth. Scandinav. *2* (1958), 149—163. — *Lund, I.*, and *K. Kristiansen:* Experiences with selective cooling of the brain. Proc. First Europ. Congr. Anaesthesiol., Wien 1962, pp. 142, 1—4. — *Løfstrøm, B.:* Induced hypothermia and intravascular aggregation. Acta anaesth. Scandinav. 1959, Suppl. 3, pp. 1—19. — *Marshall, S. B., J. C. Owens*, and *H. Swan:* Temporary circulatory occlusion to the brain of hypothermic dog. A. M. A. Arch. Surgery *72* (1956), 98—106. — *Mitchell, R. M.*, and *M. F. A. Woodruff:* The effects of local hypothermia in increasing tolerance of the kidney to ischemia. Transplant. Bull. *4* (1957), 15—17. — *Negrin, J., jr.:* A perfusion technique for regional hypothermia of the central nervous system (brain or spinal cord). Second Int. Congr. Neurol. Surg., Wash. D. C., 1961. Excerpta Medica. Int. Congr. Series No. 36, 1961, pp. 126—127. — *Negrin, J., jr.*, and *L. D. Klauber:* Direct regional hypothermia of the central nervous system: A preliminary report of a pilot project on experimental hypothermia. A. M. A. Arch. Neurol. *3* (1960), 100. — *Ommaya, A. K.*, and *M. Baldwin:* Extravascular local cooling of the brain in man. J. Neurosurg. *20* (1963), 8—19. — *Parkins, W. M., J. M. Jensen*, and *H. M. Vars:* Brain cooling in the prevention of brain damage during periods of circulatory occlusion in dogs. Ann. Surg. *140* (1954), 284—289. — *Rosomoff, H. L.:* Some effects of hypothermia on the normal and abnormal physiology of the nervous system. Proc. Roy. Soc. Med. *49* (1956), 358—364. — *Rosomoff, H. L.*, and *D. H. Holaday:* Cerebral blood flow and cerebral oxygen consumption during hypothermia. Am. J. Physiol. *179* (1954), 84—88. — *Scott, J. W., D. McQueen*, and *J. C. Callaghan:* The effect of lowered body temperature on the EEG. EEG Clin. Neurophysiol. *5* (1953), 465. — *Semb, C.:* Local cooling of the kidney for protection against operative trauma. Acta chir. Scandinav. 1959, Suppl. 245, 368—372. — *Semb, G.:* Personal communication, 1961. — *Semb, G., J. Krog*, and *K. Johansen:* Renal metabolism and blood flow during local hypothermia, studied by means of renal perfusion in situ. Acta chir. Scandinav. 1960, Suppl. 253, 196—202. — *Sweet, W. H., W. R. Brewster, P. Osgood*, and *J. C. White:* Physiology of the hypothermic state. Proc. First Int. Congr. of Neurol. Sciences, Brussels, 1957 1959, *II:* 304—311. — *Tokuoka, S., H. Aoki, K. Higashi*, and *K. Tatebayashi:* Cooling irrigation of cerebral ventricular system. Second Int. Congr. Neurol. Surg., Wash. D. C., 1961. Excerpta Medica. Int. Congr. Series, No. 36, 1961, pp. 148—149. — *White, R. J.*, and *D. E. Donald:* Selective hypothermic perfusion and circulatory arrest. Arch. Surg. *84* (1962), 292—300. — *Woodhall, R., D. H. Reynolds, S. Mahaley, jr.*, and *A. P. Sanders:* Pathologic effects of localized cerebral hypothermia. Ann. Surg. *147* (1958), 673—683.

Mayo Clinic and Mayo Foundation, Rochester, Minnesota, U.S.A.

Profound Hypothermia
and Total Circulatory Arrest in Neurosurgery:
Methods, Results, and Physiologic Effects

By

J. D. Michenfelder, A. Uihlein, C. S. MacCarty, and H. R. Terry, Jr.

With 4 Figures

Until recently hypothermia in neurosurgery had been limited to surface technics and temperatures of about 28° C; the potential hazard of ventricular fibrillation precluded further cooling. The development of extracorporeal perfusion technics has effectively circumvented this limiting factor, permitting temperatures to be lowered to 15° C and below with little additional hazard to the patient. At these temperatures the oxygen requirements are such that the brain and other vital organs can withstand total circulatory arrest for periods of 30 to 40 minutes without apparent damage.

It was our belief that periods of total circulatory arrest would be most useful as an adjunct to the surgical repair of intracranial vascular anomalies, in particular, aneurysms of the major cerebral vessels. Therefore, between March, 1960, and December, 1962, 43 patients, of which all but one had intracranial aneurysms, have been operated on at the Mayo Clinic while they were in a state of profound hypothermia and total circulatory arrest [1]—[7].

Methods

Two different technics have been used for the production of profound hypothermia. The first 18 patients in the series were cooled by means of an open-chest technic similar to that described by *Drew* [8] for cardiac surgery. In the last 25 cases, a closed-chest technic similar to that described by *Woodhall* and co-workers [9] and more recently by *Patterson* and *Ray* [10] has been used.

The anesthetic management of the patients in each group was similar. Premedication was limited to atropine, except for the occasional agitated patient who required barbiturates. Induction of anesthesia was accomplished with short-acting agents: fluothane, cyclopropane, or intravenous methohexital. The patient was then given succinylcholine (60 mg.), and tracheal intubation was performed. Anesthesia, in all patients, was maintained with fluothane in concentrations of 0.5 to 1 per cent, administered with oxygen 2 liters per minute and nitrous oxide 3 liters per minute. Patients in both groups were hyperventilated with a mechanical ventilator with positive-negative pressure phasing.

All patients were placed on blankets which could be cooled or warmed; this served a somewhat different purpose in the two groups. With the open-chest technic, the blankets were used to minimize the downward temperature drift after the patient was rewarmed; whereas, with the closed-chest technic, they were used primarily to cool the patient to 30 to 32° C before perfusion and secondarily to minimize temperature drift after rewarming. This difference in application resulted from the significantly longer cooling times necessitated by the closed-chest technic.

In the open-chest group, monitoring devices used during operations were limited to a pressure cuff, an esophageal stethoscope, and thermistors placed in the esophagus and nasopharynx. Since visual monitoring of the heart was possible, and of sufficient accuracy for clinical appraisal of the patients' cardiac status, no special monitoring devices were used, except for five patients on whom special studies were carried out [11]. In the closed-chest group, monitoring of the heart was achieved by observing central venous pressures taken by means of a catheter threaded into the superior vena cava via an antecubital vein, arterial pressures obtained by means of a needle placed in the radial artery, and the electrocardiogram monitored continuously on an oscilloscope.

Perfusion. In both technics, the conduct of the perfusion has been the responsibility of the anesthesiologist. Since the methods of cannulation and perfusion differ considerably for each technic, they will be described separately.

Open-Chest (Drew) (Fig. 1). Cannulation for this method requires a median sternotomy incision and one inguinal incision. Three cannulas are placed in the heart: one in each atrium and one, inserted through an incision in the right ventricle, in the pulmonary outflow tract. A fourth cannula is placed in an external iliac artery. Heparinization (90 mg. per square meter of body surface) is, of course, required prior to cannulation. The extracorporeal unit is primed with 3500 ml. of fresh heparinized blood; this permits rates of flow of 2.0 to 2.5 liters per minute per square meter of body surface and provides a sufficient volume for transfusion during the period of bypass.

Basically this technic bypasses both the right and left sides of the heart and permits the patient's lungs to function as oxygenators. Initially, only the left heart is bypassed, and cooling is instituted by cooling the blood in the heat exchanger to a temperature 12° C cooler than the patient's esophageal temperature. When the heart beat becomes ineffective (at 28 to 30° C), bypass of the right heart-is instituted, and cooling is continued until the temperature of the

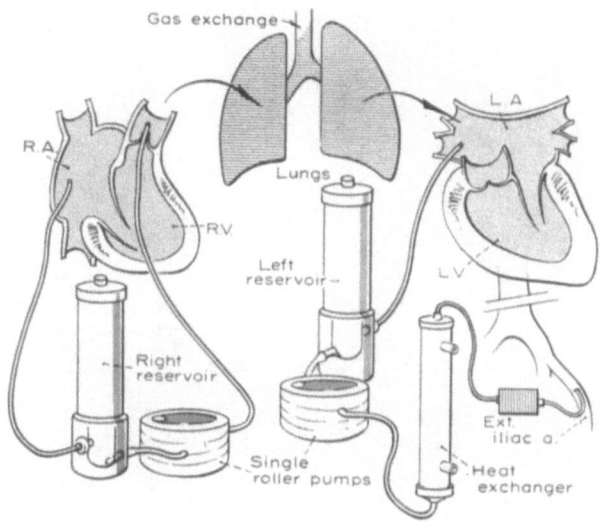

Fig. 1*. Extracorporeal circuit for open-chest technic

body is lowered to about 15° C. During cooling, repeated transfusion is required to maintain a blood flow of 2.0 to 2.5 liters per minute per square meter; this need apparently results from vasodilatation at temperatures below 28° C. (Most of the transfused blood is regained during the rewarming phase.) When the desired temperature has been achieved, either a low rate of flow of 0.6 to 1.0 liter per minute per square meter or circulatory arrest may be established for the time required by the neurosurgeon; during this time, blood is taken from the patient (about 1000 to 1500 ml.) to improve exposure and reduce stasis bleeding. When the definitive

* Figs. 1—4 are reproduced with permission from *Michenfelder, J. D., H. R. Terry, Jr., E. F. Daw, C. S. MacCarty,* and *A. Uihlein,* Profound Hypothermia in Neurosurgery: Open Versus Closed-Chest Technics. Anesthesiology. *24* (1963), 177—184.

surgical procedure has been completed, patients are rewarmed by reversing the cooling process, again maintaining a gradient of 12° C between the blood leaving the heat exchanger and the patient's esophageal temperature. When the patient's temperature reaches 30 to 32° C the heart is defibrillated and bypass of the right heart is discontinued. Bypass of the left heart is discontinued at a temperature of 37 to 38° C. The cannulas are removed and the effect of the heparin is reversed with hexadimethrine (Polybrene), 135 mg. per square meter of body surface.

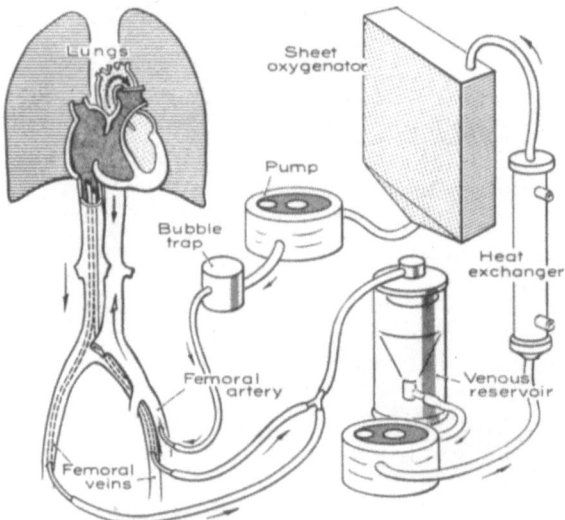

Fig. 2. Extracorporeal circuit for closed-chest technic

Closed-Chest (Fig. 2). This technic requires two inguinal incisions and three cannulas: one in each common femoral vein and one in a common femoral artery. Of the two venous cannulas, one is passed to the level of the diaphragm if possible. It is important that the venous cannulas be as large as possible.(thin-walled polyethylene cannulas with an internal diameter of 4/16 inch or 5/16 inch are satisfactory). The arterial cannula is stainless steel and has an internal diameter of 4.8 to 5.4 mm. The extracorporeal unit is a small Mayo-Gibbon pump oxygenator [12] which incorporates a Brown-Emmons heat exchanger. The volume of perfusate required for priming and transfusing during the perfusion is about 3000 ml. The perfusate consists of 1500 ml. of citrated bank blood [13] (less than 1 week old), 45 mg. of heparin, 1500 mg. of 10 per cent CaCl, 1500 ml. of 5 per cent dextrose in 0.2 per cent saline, and 240 ml.

of serum albumin. Rates of flow with this system, depending on the surface area of the patient's body, have ranged from 1.1 to 1.8 liters per minute per square meter with an average flow of 1.4 liters per minute per square meter.

Before beginning extracorporeal perfusion, the patients are cooled to 30 to 32° C on the blankets; during this time, the craniotomy and the isolation of the femoral vessels for cannulation are being carried out by two separate surgical teams. When these procedures are completed and hemostasis is adequately effected, the patient is heparinized, the cannulas are inserted, and perfusion is instituted with the rate of flow gradually increased to about 1.4 liters per minute per square meter. Cooling is again accomplished by maintaining a 12° C gradient between the temperature of the blood leaving the heat exchanger and the temperature of the esophagus. Initially, this is a partial bypass system with the heart contributing to the total-body perfusion; the part played by the heart is essential to the safety of the technic, since a rate of flow of 1.4 liters per minute per square meter would of itself be inadequate at temperatures above 28° C. At temperatures below 28°, the heart becomes ineffective and usually fibrillates; then total-body perfusion is provided by the pump-oxygenator.

During cooling, 7 per cent carbon dioxide is metered into both the lungs and the oxygenator in order to encourage cerebral vasodilatation and thereby hasten cooling of the brain [14]. Ventilation of the lungs is discontinued as soon as the heartbeat becomes ineffective. Cooling continues until a nasopharyngeal temperature of 15° C is reached, and at this point, as with the open-chest technic, either low rates of flow or circulatory arrest may be established. Rewarming is accomplished with the same rates of flow (1.1 to 1.8 liters per minute per square meter) and maintenance of a 12° C temperature gradient. When esophageal temperature reaches 26 to 28° C, the heart is defibrillated according to the technic of *Kouwenhoven* and associates [15] with a *Morris* external defibrillator. Rewarming is continued until body temperature reaches 32 to 34° C, when the cannulas are removed and Polybrene is administered. Rewarming is then continued with the blankets.

Comment. Of the two technics the closed-chest method offers the outstanding advantage of not requiring thoracotomy and cannulation of the heart. The price paid for this advantage has been primarily in terms of rates of blood flow, which are reduced to almost half those used with the open-chest method. For this reason both the cooling and the rewarming times are approximately double those of the open-chest method (Table 1); this is not thought to be a critical factor and is not a significant disadvantage. The progress of cooling and rewarming with each method is graphically demonstrated in Figs. 3 and 4. It is of interest that the rate of cooling increases in the closed-chest method after the heart fibrillates. Apparently the output of the heart resists the retrograde flow of the cold blood to the upper half of the body and when fibrillation occurs, the loss of this resistance is reflected in a sharp increase in the rate of cooling. Temperature drift during cardiac arrest and after rewarming is seen with each method, but is greater with the open-chest technic. This probably is the result of more rapid cooling and

Table 1. *Summary of Perfusion Data: Open- and Closed-Chest Technics*

	Open-chest		Closed-chest	
	Range	Mean	Range	Mean
Rates of flow (L./min./M.²)	2.0 to 2.5	2.2	1.1 to 1.8	1.4
Cooling time (minutes)	13 to 28	18	18 to 72	38
Warming time (minutes)	13 to 30	21	20 to 71	42
Low rates of flow (0.6 to 1.1 L./min./M.²) (minutes)	0 to 90	9	0 to 55	12
Cardiac arrest (minutes)	0 to 44	16	0 to 39	18

warming, which results in larger temperature gradients between the various tissues of the body. This drift has been in the range of 2 to 5° C in the open-chest group and 1 to 3° C in the closed-chest group.

The use of a dilute perfusate in the closed-chest method has reduced the amount of blood needed and has possibly improved perfusion by decreasing viscosity of the perfusate. It is reasonable to assume that a dilute perfusate and citrated bank blood would be equally applicable to the open-chest technic, but at the time that method was being used the advantages of such a system had not been appreciated. The use of 7 per cent carbon dioxide for cerebral vasodilatation is based on recent experimental work and would also apply to the open-chest technic. The reliance on external defibrillation with the closed-chest method was initially a matter of some concern, but results are so far encouraging. Of the 25 patients, 22 required defibrillation which proved difficult for only one patient, who required multiple shocks of 750 volts.

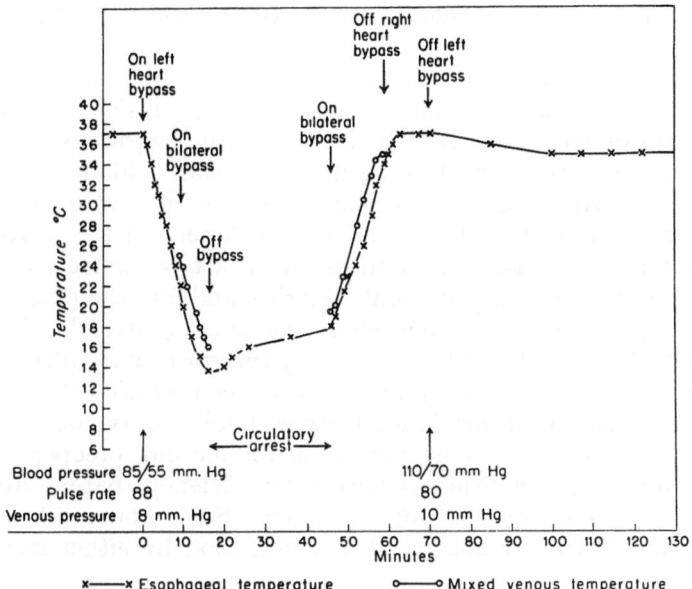

Fig. 3. Temperature graph for open-chest technic obtained from patient
with aneurysm of anterior communicating artery

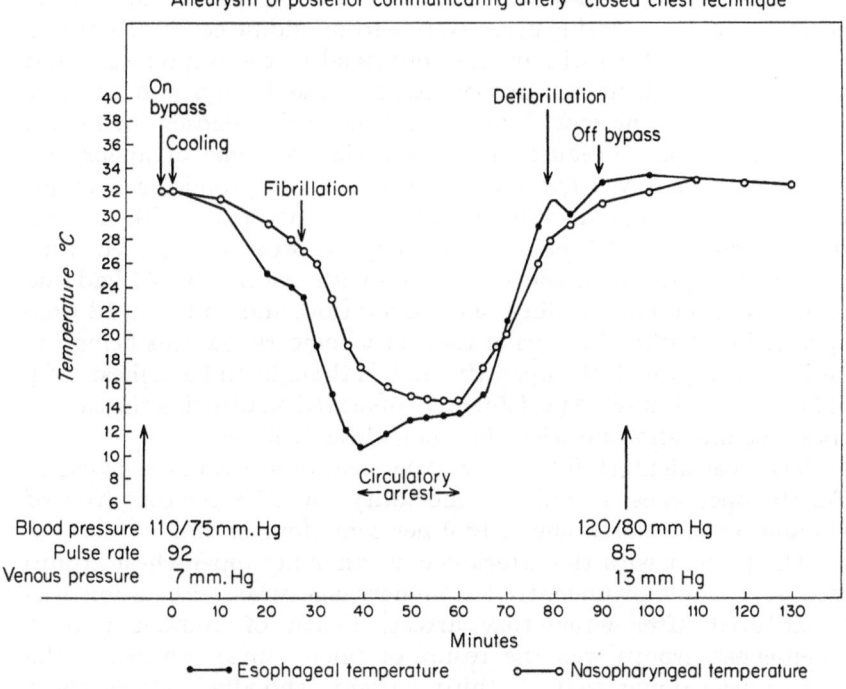

Fig. 4. Temperature graph for closed-chest technic obtained from patient
with aneurysm of posterior communicating artery

We were likewise concerned with the possibility of pulmonary vascular damage occurring during closed-chest perfusion, since there is no means of decompressing the left side of the heart while it is ineffective. To date there has been no clinical evidence of such damage occurring; however, certain measures are used to minimize this possibility, including (1) establishment of a low venous and right atrial pressure as soon as the heart is ineffective, thus minimizing flow through the right ventricle and into the pulmonary artery, (2) gradual cooling, to prevent premature ventricular fibrillation, and (3) early defibrillation during the rewarming phase. For the same reason unnecessary prolongation of perfusion during the period in which the heart is ineffective should be avoided.

With both technics it is important to rule out preoperatively such cardiac abnormalities as aortic insufficiency, patent ductus arteriosus, and coarctation of the aorta. Such abnormalities as these would obviously contraindicate perfusion by either method.

Results

Except for one patient with a large arteriovenous anomaly, all of those operated on had intracranial aneurysms. Of these, 18 arose from anterior cerebral or anterior communicating arteries, 12 from posterior communicating arteries, five from middle cerebral arteries, six from internal carotid arteries proximal to the bifurcation, and one from an ophthalmic artery. Eight patients had two or more aneurysms, the one most likely to rupture being chosen for repair.

In five cases, because of the location or type of aneurysm, definitive repair was not possible without compromising a major vessel; in these patients the aneurysm was wrapped with muscle. In the remaining 37 patients, aneurysms were obliterated with clips or by ligation. Of the 42 patients with aneurysms, 37 had one or more episodes of bleeding before operation, and, of these, 13 were operated on within 14 days of their last hemorrhage, this being the period during which the operative risk is thought to be highest [16], [17]. Twelve of these 13 patients were operated on utilizing the closed-chest technic and one with the open-chest technic.

The over-all mortality was 20.9 per cent, nine deaths in 43 cases. For the open-chest technic the mortality was 27.8 per cent (five of 18) and for the closed-chest, 16.0 per cent (four of 25).

The patient with the arteriovenous anomaly (open-chest group) died as a result of uncontrolled hemorrhage when circulation was reinstituted after circulatory arrest. Death of another patient (open-chest group) was the result of pneumonia; otherwise, the patient was doing well. A third patient who died (closed-chest group) had an infarction of the basal ganglia and internal capsule prior to operation; in retrospect this was an inoperable case. A fourth patient (closed-chest group) died of complications of a postoperative bleeding ulcer and gastrectomy; until the ulcer developed, the patient had been making an uneventful recovery. The remaining five deaths resulted from intracranial complications secondary to the repair of the vascular lesion. With the possible exception of the death from pneumonia, no deaths were attributed to the technic itself.

Table 2. *Preoperative and Postoperative Neurologic Status*

Neurologic status	Open-chest technic		Closed-chest technic	
	Preoperative (patients)	Postoperative (patients)	Preoperative (patients)	Postoperative (patients)
No deficit	8	5	10	9
Minimal deficit	6	6	6	6
Significant deficit	3	1	1	1
Mental alteration	1	1	7	5
Coma	0	0	1	0
Death	0	5	0	4

In an attempt to evaluate morbidity as well as mortality, we divided the patients into groups according to preoperative and postoperative neurologic status (Table 2). This differs somewhat from a previous classification proposed by *Botterell* and associates [16]. In the open-chest group, 14 patients had little or no preoperative deficit and four patients had significant neurologic changes. Of those who survived, 11 patients had good results and two had poor results. In the closed-chest group, 16 patients had good preoperative neurologic function and nine were severely impaired. Of those who survived, 15 had good results and six had poor results.

Comment. The results suggest that the closed-chest technic carries with it a smaller risk than does the open-chest method, although the differences in mortality and morbidity are not statistically significant because of the relatively small number of cases. This apparent difference, however, is further emphasized by the realization that 12 of the 25 in the closed-chest group were operated on within 14 days of their last hemorrhage. Thus, the over-all risk in this group was significantly greater than that of the open-chest group, wherein only one such patient was operated on.

Other factors also favor the closed-chest technic as the method of choice. By avoiding thoracotomy and thereby greatly simplifying the entire procedure, both the operative and postoperative hazards are considerably reduced. This simplification has significantly reduced the amount of blood required for the procedure from an average of 10,000 ml. for patients in the open-chest group to an average of 3900 ml. for patients in the closed-chest group. This of itself is a significant advantage, making the entire procedure more readily available and in turn reducing the potential hazard of fatal hemorrhage while the patient awaits operation. Such was the outcome in two patients during the time the open-chest method was in use.

It is of interest that during the same period that these two methods were in use, 51 other patients with intracranial aneurysms were operated on by the usual, accepted technics. In this group there were eight deaths, or an operative mortality of 15.7 per cent. However, 21 of the 51 had carotid ligation only, and 2 of these died (9.5 per cent); thus, in the group having definitive intracranial surgery (30 cases), the mortality rate was 20.0 per cent (6 deaths).

The selection of cases for profound hypothermia was, in most instances, based on the idea that the operative conditions provided by profound hypothermia and total circulatory arrest reduced to a minimum the likelihood of having to sacrifice the parent vessel in the repair of an aneurysm. Thus, in general, the patients chosen for profound hypothermia were those in whom the location or configuration of the aneurysm was such that sacrifice of the parent vessel would be likely if conventional technics were used; for example, broad-based aneurysms or aneurysms which would require considerable retraction and manipulation for exposure and repair. Also selected were those patients in whom sacrifice of a major vessel would be particularly undesirable because of an anomalous vascular configuration or the presence of multiple aneurysms involving both carotids, wherein the sacrifice of one vessel would result in increased flow in the other involved vessel.

The one major, and as yet unsolved, problem that exists with both technics for obtaining profound hypothermia is that of persistent bleeding from the operative field after circulatory arrest and rewarming. This would appear to be an inherent complication of heparinization, extracorporeal circulation, and deep hypothermia. The solution to this problem will go a long way to making this technic a more useful tool in neurosurgery, such that it would be applicable for patients with highly vascular tumors, large arteriovenous anomalies, and the like.

Table 3. *Perfusion Data in Five Cases: Open-Chest Technic**

Age, sex	Cooling time. minutes	Time of perfusion before circulatory arrest, minutes	Time of complete circulatory arrest, minutes	Time for rewarming, minutes	Total time of perfusion, minutes	Result
37, F	12	21	8	30	51	Survived
52, F	14	32	9	32	64	Survived
52, F	15	22	10	24	46	Survived
39, M	18	24	13	24	48	Survived
41, F	18	42	48	20	62	Died

* Reproduced with permission from *Rehder, Kai, J. W. Kirklin, C. S. MacCarty,* and *R. A. Theye:* Physiologic Studies Following Profound Hypothermia and Circulatory Arrest for Treatment of Intracranial Aneurysm. Ann. Surg. 156: 882—889 (Dec.) 1962. (Modified somewhat: Diagnoses and surface areas of patients were included in prior publication) [11].

Table 4. *Oxygen Uptake During Profound Hypothermia: Open-Chest Technic**

Patient	Esophageal temp., °C	$CaO_2 - CvO_2$** volume, per cent	Q,** L./min./M.²	VO_2** ml./min./M.²
1	15	1.8	1.8	32
2	13	2.1	1.1	23
3	15	1.6	1.9	30
4	16	2.1	1.4	29
5	17	2.0	1.4	28
5	17	2.0	1.4	28
6***	14	2.0	1.0	20
6***	14	2.2	1.0	22

* Reproduced with permission from *Rehder, Kai, J. W. Kirklin, C. S. MacCarty,* and *R. A. Theye:* Physiologic Studies Following Profound Hypothermia and Circulatory Arrest for Treatment of Intracranial Aneurysm. Ann. Surg. 156:882—889 (Dec.) 1962. (Modified somewhat: Title and footnotes altered.) [11].
** CaO_2 — Arterial oxygen content. CvO_2 — Venous oxygen content. Q — Flow. VO_2 — Oxygen uptake.
*** Isolated observations — no other studies carried out.

Physiologic Effects

In an attempt to determine the effect of the open-chest technic on hemodynamics and acid-base balance, special studies were carried out in five of the patients [11]. These required the preoperative placement of a cannula in the radial artery and threading of a catheter into the superior vena cava by way of an antecubital vein. Cardiac output was determined by the dye-dilution (indocyanine-green) technic [18], gases in the blood were determined by the method of *Van Slyke* and *Neill* [19], and carbon dioxide tension and buffer base were found by use of the nomogram of *Singer* and *Hastings* [20].

Pertinent perfusion data from the five cases studied are summarized in Table 3. Studies of oxygen uptake (Table 4) were carried out just prior to establishing circulatory arrest. It is of interest that the differences seen in oxygen uptake with higher blood flow rates is more than can be accounted for by the differences in temperatures

Table 5. *Hemodynamic Data: Open-Chest Technic**

Patient, time of measurement	Cardiac index (L./min./M.²)	Heart rate (beats/min.)	Stroke index (ml./M.²)	Mean right atrial pressure (mm. Hg)
1 Awake, preop.	2.5	80	32	1
Before perf.	1.8	64	29	9
After perf.	1.7	83	20	13
Awake, postop.	2.2	114	20	9
2 Awake, preop.	2.8	80	35	9
Before perf.	2.0	77	26	11
After perf.	1.7	72	24	14
Awake, postop.	2.6	96	29	—
3 Awake, preop.	3.8	73	53	1
Before perf.	2.9	64	46	16
After perf.	3.5	66	53	16
Awake, postop.	3.3	93	36	2
4 Awake, preop.	4.0	84	48	0
Before perf.	3.1	79	38	17
After perf.	2.6	75	35	19
5 Awake, preop.	3.4	88	39	—
Before perf.	2.6	88	30	15
After perf.	1.7	89	21	15

* Reproduced with permission from *Rehder, Kai, J. W. Kirklin, C. S. MacCarty*, and *R. A. Theye:* Physiologic Studies Following Profound Hypothermia and Circulatory Arrest for Treatment of Intracranial Aneurysm. Ann. Surg. 156:882—889 (Dec.) 1962. (This table constitutes an extensive abridgment of Table 3 in the publication mentioned.) [11].

at which the studies were performed. This difference is most evident between flow rates of 1.0 and 1.4 liters per minute per square meter and suggests that even at temperatures of 15° C a flow of at least 1.4 liters per minute per square meter is necessary to maintain adequate tissue perfusion.

The hemodynamic data are summarized in Table 5. The consistent drop in cardiac output after induction of anesthesia is easily accounted for by the known effects of fluothane, intermittent positive-pressure breathing, and thoracotomy. The further drop, after perfusion, is at least in part due to the fact that at this point patients' body temperatures were somewhat below normal (32 to 35° C). The return to near normal cardiac output at the end of the procedure is not accompanied by a normal stroke index and is therefore compensated for by an increase in heart rate. This consistent drop in stroke index suggests some myocardial impairment, but well within the body's normal compensatory mechanisms. In one patient these studies were repeated daily for 4 days, by which time the values obtained were all within normal limits.

Table 6. *Acid-Base Balance: Open-Chest Technic**

Patient and time of measurement		pH	PaCO$_2$** mm. Hg	BB+** mEq./L.	Vc** per cent
1 Preoperative		7.38	38	45	42
Postoperative:	Day 1	7.36	43	46	47
	Day 2	7.38	43	47	44
	Day 3	7.41	—	—	44
	Day 4	7.42	39	48	39
	Day 11	7.42	42	50	40
2 Preoperative		7.39	42	47	40
Postoperative:	Day 1	7.38	39	45	42
	Day 2	7.37	38	45	49
	Day 3	7.36	44	46	40
	Day 4	7.46	34	47	33
3 Preoperative		7.39	40	48	47
Postoperative:	Day 1	7.40	34	43	36

* Reproduced with permission from *Rehder, Kai, J. W. Kirklin, C. S. MacCarty*, and *R. A. Theye:* Physiologic Studies Following Profound Hypothermia and Circulatory Arrest for Treatment of Intracranial Aneurysm. Ann. Surg. 156:882—889 (Dec.) 1962. (This table constitutes an abridgment of Table 4 in the publication mentioned.) [11].

** PaCO$_2$: Partial pressure of carbon dioxide in arterial blood. BB+: Buffer Base. Vc: Hematocrit.

In three patients, acid-base balance was studied during the postoperative period (Table 6). The values obtained for pH, pCO$_2$, and buffer base were all within normal limits. From this it is concluded that, with adequate rates of flow, metabolic acidosis should not be considered an inherent complication of profound hypothermia but a function of the duration of circulatory arrest only.

Similar studies have been carried out on several patients operated on with the closed-chest technic [21], but as yet this work is not completed. The data so far available indicate even less disturbance in hemodynamics than was seen with the open-chest group, virtually all of the determinations falling within normal limits. Likewise, there has been no indication of pulmonary vascular damage as a result of the perfusion technic. As might be expected, because of the borderline rates of flow (1.4 liters per minute per square meter), used in the closed-chest method, we have seen a minimal but consistent metabolic acidosis in the patients studied. This has, in each instance, returned to normal by the second day and has not required any specific therapy.

Summary

Forty-three neurosurgical patients, of whom all but one had intracranial aneurysms, have been operated on at the Mayo Clinic under conditions of profound hypothermia and total circulatory arrest. Two different technics have been used to obtain these conditions: an open-chest (Drew) method requiring a median sternotomy and cannulation of the heart such that the patient's lungs can be used as the oxygenator (18 cases) and a closed-chest technic requiring peripheral cannulation of the femoral vessels and bypass through a pump-oxygenator (25 cases).

The over-all mortality was 20.9 per cent with a 27.8 per cent mortality in the open-chest group and a 16.0 per cent mortality in the closed-chest group.

The simplification permitted by the closed-chest technic favors this as the method of choice. Consideration of the mortality, morbidity, and risk also indicate this to be the preferred method.

Physiologic studies indicated minimal disturbance in hemodynamics and acid-base balance after both technics.

Zusammenfassung

43 neurochirurgische Patienten, von denen alle bis auf einen intrakranielle Aneurysmen hatten, wurden in der Mayo-Klinik unter tiefer Hypothermie und vollständigem Kreislaufstillstand operiert. Zwei verschiedene Techniken wurden hierzu angewendet: eine Methode mit eröffnetem Thorax, die eine mediane Sternotomie und eine Kanülierung des Herzens erfordert, so daß die Lunge des Patienten als Oxygenator dienen kann (18 Fälle), und eine Methode mit geschlossenem Thorax, welche eine periphere Kanülierung der Femoralgefäße und einen Bypass über einen Pump-Oxygenator voraussetzt (25 Fälle).

Die Gesamtmortalität betrug 20,9%; die der Methode mit eröffnetem Thorax 27,8% und diejenige bei geschlossenem Thorax 16,0%.

Wegen ihrer größeren Einfachheit bietet sich das Verfahren mit geschlossenem Thorax als Methode der Wahl. Auch die Vergleiche von Mortalität, Morbidität und Risiko lassen diese Methode bevorzugen.

Physiologische Untersuchungen zeigen nur geringe Störungen von Hämodynamik und Säure-Basen-Gleichgewicht nach beiden Verfahren.

Résumé

Quarante-trois malades neurochirurgicaux dont tous à part un avait un aneurysme intracranien ont été opérés à la Mayo Clinique sous hypothermie profonde et arrêt total de la circulation. Deux techniques différentes ont été utilisées pour obtenir ces conditions: Une méthode à thorax ouvert nécessitant une sternotomie médiane et canulation du cœur tel que les poumons puissent être utilisés comme oxygénateur (18 cas) et une technique à thorax fermé nécessitant une canulation des vaisseaux fémoraux et un circuit par l'oxygénateur (25 cas).

La mortalité totale fut de 20,9% avec 27,8% de mortalité dans le groupe à thorax ouvert et 16% de mortalité dans le groupe à thorax fermé.

La simplification permise par la technique à thorax fermé en fait la méthode de choix. Les considérations sur la mortalité, la morbidité, le risque aussi en font la meilleure méthode.

Des études physiologiques découvrent des troubles minimum l'équilibre hemodynamique et acide-base après ces deux techniques.

Riassunto

Quarantatre pazienti neurochirurgici, tutti portatori di aneurisma intracranico meno uno, sono stati operati alla Mayo Clinic in condizioni di ipotermia profonda e di arresto circolatorio totale. Per ottenere queste condizioni sono state usate due tecniche: una a torace aperto (Drew) che richiede una sternotomia mediana e l'incannulamento del cuore in modo da poter usare i polmoni del paziente come ossigenatore (18 casi) ed una tecnica a torace chiuso, che richiede un incannulamento periferico dei vasi femorali ed un bypass attraverso una pompa ossigenatrice (25 casi).

La mortalità totale è stata del 20,9%, il 27,8% nel gruppo a torace aperto ed il 16% in quello a torace chiuso.

La maggior semplicità permessa dalla tecnica a torace chiuso lo fa preferire all'altro. Anche le considerazioni sulla mortalità, morbilità e rischi indicano questo metodo come quello da preferirsi.

Studi fisiologici hanno mostrato come siano minimi i disturbi dell'emodenamica e dell'equilibrio acido-base dopo ambedue le tecniche.

Resumen

En la Clínica Mayo fueron operados bajo hipotermia profunda y parada total de la circulación cuarente y tres enfermos, de los cuales todos, excepto uno, tenian un aneurisma intracraneal.Fueron empleadas dos técnicas diferentes: Una con apertura del torax necesitando una esternotomiá medial y canulación de los vasos del corazón para que los pulmones pudiesen ser utilizados como oxigenador (18 casos) y otra técnica con torax cerrado que precisa de la canulación de los vasos femorales y un circuito por un oxigenador (25 casos).

La mortalidad total fué del 20,9%; con una mortalidad del 27,8 para el grupo de torax abierto y del 16% para el grupo de torax cerrado.

La simplificación que permite la técnica del torax cerrado ha hecho de este el método de elección. Las consideraciones sobre la mortalidad, morbilidad y riesgos hacen de ella el mejor método.

Los estudios fisiológicos ponen de manifiesto trastornos mínimos del equilibrio hemodinámico y acido-base después de estas dos técnicas.

References

1) *Uihlein, A., R. A. Theye, B. Dawson, H. R. Terry, Jr., D. C. McGoon, E. F. Daw*, and *J. W. Kirklin:* The Use of Profound Hypothermia, Extracorporeal Circulation and Total Circulatory Arrest for an Intracranial Aneurysm: Preliminary Report With Reports of Cases. Proc. Staff Meet., Mayo Clin. *35* (1960), 567—576. — 2) *Daw, E. F., H. R. Terry, Jr., B. Daw-*

son, and *A. Uihlein:* Repair of an Intracranial Aneurysm Using Total Body Perfusion and Profound Hypothermia: Report of a Case. Anésth. Analg. *39* (1960), 518—522. — 3) *Uihlein, A., H. R. Terry, Jr., W. S. Payne,* and *J. W. Kirklin:* Operations on Intracranial Aneurysms With Induced Hypothermia Below 15° C and Total Circulatory Arrest. J. Neurosurg. *19* (1962), 237—239. — 4) *Terry, H. R., Jr., E. F. Daw,* and *J. D. Michenfelder:* Hypothermia by Extracorporeal Circulation for Neurosurgery: An Anesthetic Technic. Anésth. Analg. *41* (1962), 241—248. — 5) *MacCarty, C. S., J. W. Kirklin,* and *A. Uihlein:* The Application of Profound Hypothermia to the Treatment of Cerebrovascular Disorders. A. Res. Nerv. Ment. Dis., Proc. (In press.) — 6) *Michenfelder, J. D., H. R. Terry, Jr., E. F. Daw, C. S. MacCarty,* and *A. Uihlein:* Profound Hypothermia in Neurosurgery: Open Versus Closed-Chest Techniques. Anesthesiology *24* (1963), 111—184. — 7) *Michenfelder, J. D., J. W. Kirklin, A. Uihlein, H. J. Svien,* and *C. S. MacCarty:* Clinical Experience With a Closed-Chest Method of Producing Profound Hypothermia and Total Circulatory Arrest in Neurosurgery. Ann. Surg. *159* (1964), 125—131. — 8) *Drew, C. E.:* Profound Hypothermia in Cardiac Surgery. Brit. M. Bull. *17* (1961), 37—42. — 9) *Woodhall, Barnes, W. C. Sealy, K. D. Hall,* and *W. L. Floyd:* Craniotomy Under Conditions of Quinidine-Protected Cardioplegia and Profound Hypothermia. Ann. Surg. *152* (1960), 37—44. — 10) *Patterson, R. H., Jr.,* and *B. S. Ray:* Profound Hypothermia for Intracranial Surgery: Laboratory and Clinical Experiences With Extracorporeal Circulation by Peripheral Cannulation. Ann. Surg. *156* (1962), 377—393. — 11) *Rehder, Kai, J. W. Kirklin, C. S. MacCarty,* and *R. A. Theye:* Physiologic Studies Following Profound Hypothermia and Circulatory Arrest for Treatment of Intracranial Aneurysm. Ann. Surg. *156* (1962), 882—889. — 12) *Kirklin, J. W.,* and *R. A. Theye:* Whole-Body Perfusion From a Pump Oxygenator for Open Intracardiac Surgery. In: *Gibbon, J. H., Jr.:* Surgery of the Chest, pp. 694—707. Philadelphia: W. B. Saunders Company. 1962. — 13) *Foote, A. V., M. Trede,* and *J. V. Maloněy, Jr.:* An Experimental and Clinical Study of the Use of Acid-Citrate-Dextrose (ACD) Blood for Extracorporeal Circulation. J. Thoracic Surg. *42* (1961), 93—109. — 14) *Payne, W. S., R. A. Theye,* and *J. W. Kirklin:* Effect of Carbon Dioxide on Rate of Brain Cooling During Conduction of Hypothermia by Direct Blood Cooling: (Unpublished data.) — 15) *Kouwenhoven, W. B., W. R. Milnor, G. G. Knickerbocker,* and *W. R. Chestnut:* Closed Chest Defibrillation of the Heart. Surgery *42* (1957), 550—561. — 16) *Botterell, E. H., W. M. Lougheed, J. W. Scott,* and *S. L. Vandewater:* Hypothermia, and Interruption of Carotid, or Carotid and Vertebral Circulation, in the Surgical Management of Intracranial Aneurysms. J. Neurosurg. *13* (1956), 1—42. — 17) *Karlsberg, P.,* and *J. E. Adams:* Value of Hypothermia and Arterial Occlusion in the Treatment of Intracranial Aneurysms. J. Neurosurg. *19* (1962), 665—674. — 18) *Theye, R. A., Kai Rehder, R. S. Quesada,* and *W. S. Fowler:* Measurement of Cardiac Output by an Indicator: Dilution Method. Anesthesiology *25* (1964), 1—4. — 19) *Van Slyke, D. D.,* and *J. M. Neill:* The Determination of Gases in Blood and Other Solutions by Vacuum Extraction and Manometric Measurement. I. J. Biol. Chem. *61* (1924), 523—573. — 20) *Singer, R. B.,* and *A. B. Hastings:* Improved Clinical Method for the Estimation of Disturbances of Acid-Base Balance of Human Blood. Medicine *27* (1948), 223—242, — 21) *Theye, R. A., J. D. Michenfelder, C. S. MacCarty,* and *J. W. Kirklin:* Physiological Studies Following the Closed-Chest Technic of Profound Hypothermia and Total Circulatory Arrest in Neurosurgery. (Unpublished data.)

III. Hypothermia as a Therapeutic Procedure

Clinique de Neurochirurgie — Hôpital de Purpan — Toulouse (France)

Moderate Hypothermia in Cranio-Cerebral Trauma

By

G. Lazorthes and L. Campan

Moderate hypothermia can be defined as reduction of body temperature to levels above 30° C (rectal). It differs physiologically and technically from the deep hypothermia of vascular surgery using temperatures lower than 27° C. Moderate hypothermia obviates the risk of ventricular fibrillation, it is easier to achieve and can be prolonged for one or several days. Its effect in lowering metabolism and protecting the brain are less but its applications are wider, especially in cranio-cerebral trauma.

Though the use of moderate hypothermia began more than twenty years ago, following the initial work of *Temple Fay* (1941), more than the mere lapse of time is required to establish the value of a method. Although many people took it up enthusiastically, it was not adopted generally and this may have been due to its complexity. It continues to evoke interesting discussions, particularly since the work of *Laborit* (1952) gave it a new impetus and direction. That is why it is on our agenda in 1963 as it was on that of the International Congress in Brussels in 1957 and of the meeting of the Neurosurgical Society of the French Language in 1961. Even if agreement is reached on its theoretical value, this is far from so concerning its applications, technique and even its degree of efficiency.

Mode of Action

With moderate hypothermia a reduction of cerebral metabolism can be expected, and, as a result of this, an increase of the cerebral resistance to anoxia is produced and also an increased tolerance to various types of local injury (traumatic, operative, haemorrhagic, malacic) productive of perifocal ischaemia. It can also be expected to reduce cerebral swelling (haemodynamic swelling and true oedema), to balance cerebral haemodynamics and, finally, to inhibit the endocrinal vegetative reactions to injury. All these objectives can be achieved to some extent.

Indications

A fundamental principle follows from the work of *Rosomoff*: the efficacy of hypothermia depends on its early application. It is

as easy to prevent the appearance of an acute vegetative syndrome
when its appearance seems inevitable as it is difficult to reverse it
once it has become established.

This idea would lead one to pessimistic conclusions. If hypothermia during operation stands a good chance of ameliorating complications, its use in trauma poses a difficult problem since head injuries
are sent to us, more often than not, in a state of vegetative dys-
function already established for several hours if not several
days.

Many of the failures of hypothermia in cerebral trauma result
from its having been started too late, after lesions and reactions
have set in, and ended too early, before the disappearance of these
reactions and stabilisation of lesions.

Yet it is in cerebral trauma that hypothermia has its most important indications. Brain injury produces immediately, or very
quickly, inaccessible lesions which are most probably in the brainstem. That is to say in the vegetative areas and the reticular formation. It is probable that shearing stress and stretching of the
branches of the Circle of Willis supplying the hypothalamus is
responsible for these immediate lesions (*Gillingham*, 1954; *Lazorthes*
et al., 1956). Since it is impossible to know from the very beginning
the severity and reversibility of these lesions, assessing the value of
any therapeutic method will be uncertain. It is useless to hope that
hypothermia will improve necrosis already present. At most one
may hope to limit its spread, prevent the formation of secondary
lesions, increase the tolerance of vulnerable nervous areas and
moderate the reactive syndrome.

Its greatest chance of being effective, if the damage is not fatal,
lies in its being applied early enough. *Wertheimer* believes that it
must be started within three hours of injury. Later, its practical
effects are less, though it is still capable of prolonging
survival.

The application and maintenance of hypothermia in trauma
presents greater difficulties than in ordinary neurosurgery or in
general surgery. The first difficulty is apparent at the outset. It is as
easy to lower the temperature of a normothermic subject as it is
difficult to overcome a hyperthermia which has already set in and
is increasing. When agitation and respiratory difficulties are also
present the problem becomes even more difficult. New difficulties
are encountered when it is necessary to prolong hypothermia beyond
three or four days. It would often be desirable to prolong hypothermia beyond this time but this is practically impossible from the
technical point of view.

Techniques

The techniques of hypothermia have been modified little since the Congress at Brussels in 1957. Controversy still continues on one important point: is it better to obtain hypothermia by simple cooling or by cooling in association with neuroplegia? As far as we are concerned we have followed the second method since 1952.

The physical methods of cooling, whether they are internal or external (through conduction, convection or radiation), have all serious inconveniences if they are used without previous preparation. The organism struggles against the cold before allowing its temperature to fall. The phase of "narcosis by cold", which is theoretically attained at 30° C and at which we aim, is always preceded by a sympatheticotonic phase when the organism defends itself by vasoconstriction, by mobilising hepatic glycogen and by activating the pituitary, adrenal and thyroid glands. Hypothermia would never have become a therapeutic method if means had not been available to lessen the disorders which this initial phase involves.

Lowered metabolism, ideally, should not only be shown by a diminution of tissue oxygen consumption but also, and more importantly, by a diminution of the products of metabolism, notably of fixed acids.

Two methods have been proposed for preventing the phase of reaction: narcosis and neuroplegia.

Narcosis is a simple procedure for obtaining sensory and motor tranquillity in the course of the initial phase of the reaction.

It may be objected, however, that it masks the reactions rather than suppresses them. In fact, some alarming biological signs are apparent at the start of cooling under narcosis. Hyperazotaemia, hyperglycaemia, a diminution of glycogen reserves or an eosinopenia giving evidence of the reaction to injury.

H. Laborit has frequently pointed out that general anaesthetics, and notably the barbiturates, easily lower the consumption of oxygen without lowering metabolic level or its products to the same extent.

Moreover, narcosis is technically ill-suited to prolonged hypothermia. It is inadequate for the comatose and consequently for the whole field of cerebral trauma.

Neuroplegia. In 1951 we proposed the association of neuroplegia and cooling in neurosurgery, which had been introduced a short time before by *H. Laborit* for use in general surgery under the name of artificial hibernation.

It seems to be suitable for brief hypothermia during operations (in association with analgesics) and it is even more suitable for hypothermia of longer duration. It can even be applied to the comatose.

Two factors justify its use. It alone possesses a certain effectiveness against the disturbances of function in brainstem damage. Moreover, in our opinion, it makes the application of hypothermia easier than does narcosis. Is it not logical after all to use anti-adrenaline substances to prevent the sympatheticotonic phase ?

The number of neuroplegic and neuroleptic substances has increased in the course of the past five years. Apart from the major derivatives of phenothiazine (chlorpromazine and levomepromazine) and its allied products (chlorprotixine) we also have minor derivatives, allied to the tranquillisers. We can also add the group of butyrophenones. Hydergin and procaine are still of the same interest. We have previously investigated the properties of these drugs. They form a fairly substantial group from which we can, in each case, choose the most appropriate substances for their effects on consciousness, on general and cerebral haemodynamics, on respiration and on the whole of the vegetative functions.

Neuroplegia cannot escape all criticism and *D. Vovet* has pointed out that it forms a "chemical scalpel" requiring very delicate handling.

In a recent paper *P. E. Maspes* (1962) pointed out that neuroplegics do not on their own lower the metabolic rate of the organism and this could raise doubts as to their use as aids to cooling. We have endeavoured to answer this objection in advance. It is generally the case that the most powerful neuroplegics if used alone and in less than toxic doses are not absolute hypometabolising agents (there is only one absolute agent: hypothermia) but are, as it were eumetabolic agents. They do not lower metabolism below the basal level, they only inhibit metabolic increases from sympatheticotonus, hyperthyroidism and agitation. What must be expected from them is this, that they contribute to maintaining the organism in the optimal metabolic condition whatever injury it has sustained. Is not such a normalisation a good preparation for hypothermic hypometabolism ?

P. E. Maspes also considers that neuroplegics are devoid of anti-stress action. This is a difficult problem. The concept of stress is so complex that one cannot see how to define an anti-stress drug with precision. In any case it seems that the neuroplegics have a favourable effect on several elements of stress, such as have been analysed by *H. Selye*. *G. Tardieu* and his collaborators (who, however, have not completely accepted *H. Laborit*'s theories) consider that chlorpromazine is capable of inhibiting histological manifestations of the Neilly syndrome of irritation. The preventive anti-shock action of the neuroplegics has today been proved by more than ten years of surgical experience in France and elsewhere.

Neuroplegia is blamed for depressing respiration. This is not a real danger. Nothing in the pharmacodynamics nor in the use of neuroplegics is suspect in this respect. If respiratory depression has been observed in neuroplegic patients, it is certain that it was not due to the neuroplegics but to associated substances, narcotics or morphine. It is true that the latter are often abused. Overdosage by morphine is easily corrected by mechanical respiration on the one hand or by morphine antidotes on the other.

In our view the criticism levelled at the depressive effects on circulation of the major neuroplegics and even of hydergine, should be taken very seriously. As has been seen they are powerful vaso-dilators and their overdosage can cause collapse of blood pressure. Hypotensive patients and, even more, those who are hypertensive, are extremely sensitive in this respect. Even low doses at times bring about a serious collapse in patients who have intracranial hyper-tension. We have pointed out this danger repeatedly.

This criticism, however, is levelled less at the remedies than at the method of using them. The dosology of neuroplegics is individual. Their administration must be in divided doses, spaced out and in suitable dilution and always under blood pressure control. The use of standardised doses is not to be recommended in neurosurgery.

J. LeBeau (1954) in France and P. E. Maspes (1962) in Italy consider that neuroplegia depresses consciousness, especially in the case of cranial trauma. This criticism is partially justified. At first sight it is very unsatisfactory to administer hypnogogues to an unconscious patient. It is, however, even less satisfactory to ad-minister narcotics as certain detractors of neuroplegics are in the habit of doing. The present range of neuroplegics admits of an ade-quate choice of substances. Hydergine associated with procaine or xylocaine is harmless in deep comas. After more than ten years of widespread use it is, moreover, generally accepted that the least controversial effect of neuroplegia is to prolong survival of those seriously injured. That is to say that it does not aggravate the coma.

The same authors think that neuroplegia masks vegetative signs and even neurological signs and thereby makes clinical supervision more difficult. This criticism, which recognises at least the sympto-matic efficiency of neuroplegia, does not seem justified according to P. Wertheimer and J. Descotes. On the contrary, by the calm it brings about neuroplegia facilitates electrical and angiographic investigations. After all, if it merits this criticism, hypothermia deserves it even more since at about 32° C a real symptomatic extinction results.

Results

The good results of hypothermia used during operation are generally admitted. The ease of operating, the reduction of cerebral swelling and the reduction of complications are agreed. Operations involving a risk of brainstem damage always benefit from hypothermia, which is easy to achieve under neuroplegia and analgesia, and even more so under narcosis, and this can be continued in the post-operative phase.

By contrast the use of hypothermia in cerebral trauma is still an open question. In this sphere the results must be considered with extreme caution. Three types of result must be considered: the immediate symptomatic results, definitive effects on mortality and the way in which hypothermia modifies the evolution of the injury.

Immediate symptomatic improvement is denied by no one. In too many cases, however, the optimism of the first few days is replaced by disappointment later at the stage of re-warming, which is accompanied by a recurrance of all the symptoms. As it is not possible to carry out hypothermia for more than three or four days, there is a tendency to substitute for it, neuroplegia pure and simple. Many patients die at this stage. It is not uncommon, however, to obtain a progressive improvement in the vegetative state. Often the clinical picture ends by running a subacute course.

All authors admit that the efficacy of hypothermia in the vegetative syndrome during the first three of four days after injury is encouraging. Many believe that neuroplegia contributes largely to this result.

If one considers, however, the overall mortality, the figures are less encouraging. They show the following mortality rates: with simple hypothermia: 41% (*Lewin*, 1957), 43% (*Sedzmir*, 1959), and 68% (*Maspes*, 1962). With neuroplegia and hypothermia: 53% (*Wertheimer*, 1957), 70% for ourselves (1957), and 84% for *Woringer*, though his figures date back as far as 1954. A comparison between the two methods, if one can admit its validity, is in favour of hypothermia without neuroplegia.

Nevertheless the figures which have been published still indicate a positive balance. In the figures we put forward in 1957, we only took into account those who were seriously and, as we thought, fatally injured. We recorded 28% of survivals, which seemed to us a significant number. This figure is, however, one of the least good of all the results published.

The analysis of our personal figures shows that hypothermia has contributed by modifying the evolution of post-traumatic morbidity. Before 1952 the greater number of those injured died in the first few days in a fully established vegetative state. The position changed from the moment we started using hypothermia with neuroplegia. Twenty-one per cent of our injured patients died within a few hours of treatment, possibly as a result of imperfections in the first phase of hypothermia. Only 6.3% died during hypothermia (with an average duration of three days) after having appeared to benefit from it. 21% died during the stage of re-warming or during the next two days. 23% died during the course of the next few weeks in a precarious subacute state dominated by complex disturbances of consciousness, by hydrogen-ion and irremedial metabolic disturbances and by infectious complications. 28% survived.

What follows from these figures ? The period of lowest mortality coincides with the period of hypothermia which must be considered a measure of protection during the evolution of morbidity after injury. It is preceded and followed by two critical periods of high mortality, the cooling stage and the stage of re-warming. However, it does allow a greater number of head injuries to pass through the acute phase and to reach this secondary phase where the chances of survival increase daily. It is true that this survival has more than once been overshadowed by bad neurological sequelae which the nature of the established lesions has made inevitable. But recoveries with good neurological status are becoming more and more common.

Conclusions

1) Moderate hypothermia does not seem to involve any serious hazard, whatever method is employed. This was the opinion of the French Society of Neurosurgery in 1962.

2) The general indication for hypothermia is in the prophylaxis and treatment of the syndrome of brainstem damage.

3) Hypothermia improves operative conditions in major neurosurgery and helps the later post-operative stages. It has made it possible to extend the indications for operation. In cerebral trauma there is no doubt of its symptomatic efficacy and it has very probably contributed to lowering the mortality.

4) The part played by neuroplegia in hypothermia is still controversial. We ourselves, like many authors in France, support its use. We agree with *Wertheimer* that the part played by neuroplegia should not be underestimated.

5) The difficulties of supervising patients under hypothermia, especially under prolonged hypothermia, are considerable. This

necessitates constant supervision and also controls only possible in resuscitation units. Attempts to apply hypothermia without these controls involve a risk. Such attempts have occasioned many of the failures in this most interesting of methods and much of the caution with which it has been treated.

6) Hypothermia has, for a long time, seemed the most heroic means at our disposal in the struggle against the acute neuro-vegetative syndrome. This is no longer so today. It takes its place with many other treatments: in the first place that of respiratory resuscitation, going, if necessary, as far as tracheostomy and mechanically controlled respiration, followed by the treatment of circulatory resuscitation, treatment of cerebral oedema, and adjustment of acid-base balance. All these treatments are inter-related and it is difficult to tell the part which each plays in the whole field of neurosurgical resuscitation.

Summary

The conclusion of the meeting of the Neurosurgical Society of the French Language in 1962 was: "Moderate hypothermia seems to involve no severe risk, whatever the method used to achieve it. Moderate hypothermia can be obtained by a combination of general anaesthetics, neuroplegics, and external refrigeration."

This is our conclusion also, except that anaesthetics are nearly always undesirable in severe trauma.

1) The general indication for hypothermia is in the prophylaxis of the reactive syndrome associated with very severe cerebral lesions. This reaction is called by several names: acute neuro-vegetative syndrome, severe generalised irritation syndrome (G. Tardieu) or brainstem lesion syndrome.

2) Hypothermia improves the post-operative condition and lessens sequelae in major neurosurgery and thereby increases the indications for surgery. In cerebral trauma its symptomatic efficacy is obvious and it very probably contributes to a reduction the mortality.

3) The contribution of neuroplegia to hypothermia is always in question. We continue to use this method as do many others in France. We are of the same opinion as Wertheimer who says: "it is useless to discriminate between the part played by neuroplegia and by cooling."

4) The difficulties of supervising the patient under hypothermia, especially when prolonged, are considerable. Constant supervision by the presence of medical personnel is necessary as well as the monitoring of various functions which can only be carried out

in resuscitation services. To start hypothermia without such monitoring is really hazardous.

5) For a long time hypothermia for combatting the neurovegetative syndrome seemed to be a heroic measure. This attitude is now changed and it merely takes its places amongst a number of suchlike measures. Respiratory resuscitation is the most urgent need and tracheostomy and mechanically controlled respiration should be used if necessary. Following this, restoration of circulation and blood pressure should be achieved, cerebral oedema treated and hydrogen-ion and metabolic deviations corrected. All these treatments are closely related and it is impossible to define the precise part played by each in the overall efficiency of neurosurgical resuscitation.

Zusammenfassung

Die Schlußfolgerung des Kongresses 1962 der „Société de Neurochirurgie de Langue Française" lautete, daß „die mäßige Hypothermie kein größeres Risiko bedeutet, welche Methode der Ausführung auch immer angewendet wird. Diese mäßige Hypothermie kann erreicht werden durch die Kombination von allgemeinen Anästhetica, Neuroplegica und äußere Abkühlung". Das ist auch unsere Schlußfolgerung, allerdings mit der Einschränkung, daß bei schweren Verletzungen Anästhetica fast immer kontraindiziert sind.

1. Die allgemeine Indikation zur Hypothermie ist in der Prophylaxe und Therapie der reaktiven Veränderungen zu sehen, die den sehr schweren Hirngewebsläsionen folgen und die man mit verschiedenen Namen bezeichnet: akutes neurovegetatives Syndrom, schweres allgemeines Irritations-Syndrom (*G. Tardieu*) oder axiales Schädigungs-Syndrom.

2. Hypothermie verbessert die Operationsbedingungen und -folgen in der großen Neurochirurgie. Sie hat es ermöglicht, die Indikationen zur Tumorentfernung zu erweitern. Bei den Hirnverletzungen ist ihre symptomatische Wirksamkeit unbestritten. Sie hat mit großer Wahrscheinlichkeit dazu beigetragen, die Mortalität zu mindern.

3. Die Anwendung der Neuroplegica bei der Hypothermie ist immer noch umstritten. Wir sind, wie die meisten französischen Autoren, Anhänger ihrer Verwendung. Wir teilen die Ansicht von *Wertheimer*, „daß es unsinnig ist, die Bedeutung der Neuroplegica oder der Abkühlung herabzusetzen".

4. Die Schwierigkeiten der Pflege des Patienten sind in Hypothermie, und besonders in langdauernder Hypothermie, sehr groß. Sie verlangen ständige Anwesenheit und Kontrollen, wie sie sich nur in Wiederbelebungszentren verwirklichen lassen, Versuche, die Hypothermie ohne diese Voraussetzungen durchzuführen, bedingen ein Risiko. Von daher erklären sich manche Versager und Ablehnungen dieser interessanten Methode.

5. Die Hypothermie schien lange Zeit die heroischste Waffe zu sein, über die wir im Kampf gegen die akuten neurovegetativen Syndrome verfügen. Heute ist es nicht mehr so. Sie hat ihren Platz unter zahlreichen anderen Behandlungsverfahren gefunden: an erster Stelle steht die Sicherung der Atmung, bis hin zur Tracheotomie und künstlichen Beatmung; es folgen die Maßnahmen zur Stabilisierung des Kreislaufs, die Behandlung des Hirn-

184 G. Lazorthes and L. Campan:

ödems und der Ausgleich von Störungen der Elektrolytbalance. Alle diese Maßnahmen gehören zusammen, so daß es schwierig geworden ist, für eine einzelne davon genau festzulegen, welche Wirksamkeit sie im Gesamt der neurochirurgischen Wiederbelebung hat.

Résumé

La conclusion de la réunion de la Société de Neurochirurgie de Langue Française en 1962 fut que „l'hypothermie modérée parait ne comporter aucun péril grave, quelle que soit la méthode utilisée pour la réaliser. Cette hypothermie modérée peut être obtenue par l'association d'anesthésiques généraux, de neuroplégiques et de la réfrigération extérieure". C'est aussi notre conclusion, à cette réserve près que les anesthésiques sont presque toujours à proscrire en traumatologie grave.

1. L'indication générale de l'hypothermie réside dans la prophylaxie et le traitement du syndrome réactionnel lié aux lésions cérébrales gravissimes que l'on désigne sous des noms divers: syndrome neuro-végétatif aigu, syndrome d'irritation généralisée grave (G. *Tardieu*) ou syndrome de souffrance axiale.

2. L'hypothermie améliore les conditions et les suites opératoires en neurochirurgie majeure. Elle a permis d'étendre les indications d'exérèses. En traumatologie cérébrale son efficacité symptomatique n'est pas douteuse et elle a très probablement contribué à diminuer la mortalité.

3. La participation de la neuroplégie à l'hypothermie est toujours discutée. Nous en sommes, quant à nous, partisans comme beaucoup d'auteurs en France. Nous partageons l'avis de *Wertheimer* selon qui „il est inutile de discriminer la part qui revient à la neuroplégie ou au refroidissement".

4. Les difficultés de la surveillance du sujet en hypothermie (en hypothermie prolongée surtout) sont assez considérables. Elle nécessite une présence permanente et des contrôles seulement réalisables dans les services de ranimation. Les tentatives de mise en hypothermie faites en dehors de ces moyens de contrôle comportent un risque. De là bien des échecs d'une méthode des plus intéressante et bien des réticences à son égard.

5. L'hypothermie a paru être longtemps le moyen le plus héroïque dont nous disposions pour lutter contre le syndrome neurovégétatif aigu. Il n'en va plus de même aujourd'hui. Elle prend rang parmi de nombreuses autres thérapeutiques: en première urgence les thérapeutiques de ranimation respiratoire allant s'il le faut jusqu'à la trachéotomie et à la respiration contrôlée mécanique, ensuite les thérapeutiques de ranimation circulatoire, les thérapeutiques anti-œdème cérébrale, l'équilibration métabolique hydroionique. Toutes ces thérapeutiques sont étroitement corrélatives et il est devenu bien difficile de préciser la part qui revient à chacune dans l'efficacité globale de la ranimation neurochirurgicale.

Riassunto

La conclusione del Meeting della Società di Neurochirurgia dei Paesi di Lingua Francese è stata: „L'ipotermia moderata non sembra avere eccessivi rischi, qualunque sia il metodo usato per ottenerla. L'ipotermia moderata può essere ottenuta con l'associazione di anestetici generali, di neuroplegici e con il raffreddamento esterno."

Questa è anche la nostra conclusione, se si eccettuano gli anestetici, che sono quasi sempre da non usare nei traumi gravi.

1. L'applicazione generale dell'ipotermia nella profilassi e nel trattamento della sindrome reazionale è legata alle più gravi lesioni cerebrali chiamate con diversi nomi: sindrome acuta neuro-vegetativa, irritazione grave generalizzata, sindrome delle lesioni assiale.

2. L'ipotermia migliora le condizioni e le sequele delle operazioni neurochirurgiche più gravi. Essa permette di estendere le indicazioni dell'exeresi.

Nella traumatologia cerebrale la sua efficacia sintomatica è ovvia e molto probabilmente contribuisce a ridurre la mortalità.

3. Il contributo della neuroplegia all'ipotermia è sempre stato discusso. Per parte nostra noi siamo convinti dell'utilità di questo metodo, come del resto molti autori in Francia. Noi siamo dell'opinione di *Wertheimer* secondo il quale ,,é inutile discriminare la parte che appartiene alla neuroplegia da quella che appartiene al raffreddamento".

4. Le difficoltà di sorveglianza del paziente in ipotermia (soprattutto nell'ipotermia prolungata) sono molto considerevoli. Essa richiede una presenza costante e controlli che sono solamente possibili in servizi di rianimazione. I tentativi di iniziare l'ipotermia senza questi mezzi di controllo sono sempre pericolosi.

5. Per lungo tempo l'ipotermia sembrava il mezzo più eroico a disposizione contro la sindrome neurovegetativa acuta. Oggi è molto diverso. Essa prende il suo posto insieme a molte altre terapie. In ordine di urgenza è preceduta dalla terapia di rianimazione respiratoria, e se necessario della tracheotomia, e della respirazione meccanica controllata, poi dalla terapia di rianimazione cardiocircolatoria, dalla terapia antiedema cerebrale e da quella per mantenere il bilancio idro-ionico. Tutte queste terapie sono intimamente correlate ed è difficile precisare la parte che riguarda ognuna di esse nell'efficienza globale della rianimazione neurochirurgica.

Resumen

En la reunión de la Sociedad de Neurocirugía de Lengua Francesa de 1962 se llegó a la conclusión que la hipotermia moderada no parece ocasionar ningún peligro grave, cualquiera que sea el método empleado para realizarla. Esta hipotermia moderada puede obtenerse mediante la asociación de anestesia general, neuroplégicos y refrigeración externa. Esta es también la conclusión a que hemos llegado nosotros, salvo en los casos traumaticos graves en los cuales los anestésicos están casi siempre contraindicados.

1. La indicación general de la hipotermia radica en la profilaxis y tratamiento del síndrome reaccional que acompaña a las graves lesiones cerebrales y designado bajo los nombres diversos de: síndrome neuro-vegetativo agudo, síndrome de irritación generalizada grave (*G. Tardieu*) ó síndrome de sufrimiento axial.

2. La Hipotermia mejora las condiciones y el curso post-operatorio de la neurocirugía mayor. Ha permitido ampliar las indicaciones de exéresis. En traumatología cerebral su eficacia sintomática es evidente y ella ha contribuido probablemente a disminuir la mortalidad.

3. La participación de la neuroplegia en la hipotermia siempre es objeto de discusión. En lo que se refiere a nosotros somos partidarios, como muchos autores en Francia. Compartimos la opinión de *Wertheimer* que dice que ,,es ínútil tratar de discriminar que parte corresponde a la hipotermia ó al enfriamiento".

4. Las dificultades para la vigilancia del enfermo bajo hipotermia (en hipotermia prolongada sobre todo) son bastante considerables. Necesita de vigilancia permenente y controles solamente realizables en los servicios de reanimación. Las tentativas de efectuar hipotermias fuera de estos métodos de control llevan un grave riesgo. Esta es la causa de muchos fracasos de uno de los métodos más interesantes y de muchas reticencias respecto al mismo.

5. La hipotermia pareció ser durante mucho tiempo el medio más heroico del cual disponiamos para luchar contra el síndrome neurovegetativo agudo. Hoy dia no ocurre lo mismo. Tiene su lugar entre otras numerosas terapéuticas: de primera urgencia las terapéuticas de reanimación respiratoria que van en caso necesario desde la traqueotomía hasta la respiración mecánica controlada, después las terapéuticas de reanimación circulatoria, las terapéuticas anti-edema cerebral, el equilibrio metabólico hidroiónico. Todas estas terapéuticas están estrechamente unidas y resulta muy difícil precisar la parte que corresponde a cada una de ellas en la eficacia global de la reanimación neuroquirúrgica.

References

Laborit, H.: L'hypothermie dans le traitement des traumatismes cranio-encéphaliques. Agressologie 1963, IV, 1 (encart). — *Laborit, H.,* et *P. Huguenard:* Pratique de l'hibernothérapie, pp. 136—180. Paris: Ed. Masson et Cie. 1934. — *Lazorthes, G.,* et *L. Campan:* L'hypothermie dans le traitement des traumatismes crânio-cérébraux. 1er Congrès International de clinique hémologique, Bruxelles, Juillet 1957. — *Lazorthes, G.,* et *L. Campan:* Hypothermia in the treatment of cranio cerebral traumatism. J. Neurosurg. *15* (1958), 162—167. — *Le Beau, J., J. Gruner* et *P. Minuit:* Remarques sur une série de 400 traumatismes crânio-cérébraux graves. Neurochirurgie *1955,* I, 1, 117—126. — *Lewin, W.:* Planning for head injury. Brit. Med. J. 1959, 17 Jan., *1,* 131. — *Rosomoff, H. L.:* Hypothermia and cerebral vascular lesions. Experimental interruption of the middle cerebral artery during hypothermia. J. Neurosurg. *13* (1956), 244—255. — *Rosomoff, H. L.:* Experimental brain injury and delayed hypothermia. Surg. Gyn. Obst. *1960,* 110, I, 27—32. — *Wertheimer, P.,* and *J. Descotes:* Traumatologie crânienne. Paris: Ed. Masson et Cie. 1961. (This book contains the essentials of the bibliography.) — *Wertheimer, P.:* L'hypothermie en neurochirurgie. Paris: Ed. Masson et Cie. 1963. — Consult also: Comptes-rendus du 1er Congrès International de Neurochirurgie, 1957, éd. „Acta Medica Belgica" Bruxelles.

Clinica Neurochirurgica — Università degli Studi — Milano (Italy)

Final Remarks on the Clinical Use of Hypothermia in Neurosurgery

By

P. E. Maspes

I am going to summarize briefly the conclusions we have reached about indications and use of hypothermia in neurosurgery, but first I would like to thank all the distinguished reporters to this Symposium. Their important original contributions enable us to make a valuable up to date review of the problems concerning the systemic and neurological pathophysiology of the hypothermic state, the clinical indications of hypothermia and the various techniques of anaesthesia.

Thanks to their reports we now know that many problems have been or are going to be solved, whereas new work is waiting, especially in the field of hypothermic cellular metabolism.

We can now believe that the use of hypothermia in neurosurgery rests on sound theoretical and clinical grounds and that the new method is now well documented. This statement is surely true for moderate hypothermia whereas we have to withold our judgement on profound hypothermia and on selective brain cooling.

Dealing first with the surgical use of *moderate hypothermia* I can say that our opinion comes from the results reported in the literature and from our personal experience which is based on over 200 cases.

The reports in the literature are actually not always useful because many data are not really pertinent and often not elaborated statistically. We have therefore tried to elaborate our data following statistical rules.

The following conclusions will reflect our personal opinion which however may not be final.

Moderate hypothermia if used with correct indications and performed by a qualified team, is not dangerous *per se* even in old or hypertensive patients.

We believe that the main indication for the use of hypothermia in neurosurgery is direct intracranial attack on aneurysms of the large vessels of the base of the brain. We think that moderate hypothermia can offer real advantages for the radical treatment of these aneurysms since, with interruption of the cerebral blood flow, it allows in a higher number of cases, safe dissection and ligature of the aneurysmal sac. Moreover in many cases hypothermia helps to prevent intraoperative rupture of the sac and when this has occurred, it reduces the dangers of the accident, allowing the surgeon to deal with the situation more calmly and with safety.

We also come to the conclusion that besides the advantages connected with total or partial cerebral blood flow interruption, moderate hypothermia does not generally provide marked protection against surgical trauma and does not improve the final outcome in cases of aneurysms operated in coma, shortly after bleeding.

We believe that although sometimes proved, protection against vascular spasm is not always present.

As for the use of moderate hypothermia in the surgery of particularly dangerous tumors because of their vascularization or for their vicinity to brain stem centers, on the basis of a comparison between two groups of statistically comparable patients, we conclude that hypothermia does not provide here substantial advantages either for postoperative course or for the final outcome. We however have to withhold our judgement on some particular tumors such as craniopharyngiomas. We cannot make a statement on these tumors because our series and those reported by others are not yet sufficiently large. We can however say that hypothermia seemed to us to protect these cases against endocrinologic postoperative disturbances.

We do not think that moderate hypothermia is strictly indicated in the surgical treatment of arteriovenous malformations but it can be very useful in some selected cases when the interruption of the blood flow becomes necessary.

As for the other surgical advantages which could be provided by the use of moderate hypothermia, such as decreased dural tension and reduced blood flow, we conclude from our study that these effects are usually present but irrelevant and, being more easily obtained by other means, do not alone justify the use of hypothermia.

The conclusion reached at the 1961 French Symposium on hypothermia at Montpellier, on the use of *profound hypothermia* with circulatory arrest, in neurosurgery, was mainly negative. It has however now to be pointed out that at that meeting nobody could refer to a large experience in this field. We now have a great amount of data, coming from Dr. *Uihlein*'s group, which has the facilities provided by the Mayo Clinic organization.

These data show that deep hypothermia, if properly performed by a particularly trained team, does not *per se* imply any special risk for the nervous system, but has only those connected to the technique of extracorporeal circulation and mainly to the bleeding from the operative field when blood flow is resumed.

From the data reported by these authors we cannot however see for deep cooling any other particular indication besides those already mentioned for moderate hypothermia. I believe we can conclude here that this difficult, complicated and expensive method, is only indicated in some exceptional cases which require continuous interruption of circulation for periods over 20 minutes.

Considering now *selective cooling*, we can say that it has now enough experimental grounds to justify its clinical use.

Among the largest series to date is the one presented by Prof. *Kristiansen* and his group, who operated on 27 patients using selective cerebral hypothermia, cooling blood taken from the carotid and giving it back through the same vessel at the neck. According to these authors A-V malformations are the more suitable cases for this technique. The method seems stimulating. We think however that it cannot as yet be considered safe enough to be included in the current practice. The reasons are:

a) a team trained to extracorporeal circulation is required;

b) stopping the perfusion does not allow such a complete arrest of intracranial blood flow as it can be obtained by clamping the four vessels at the neck;

c) as with other methods of extracorporeal circulation, postoperative technical complications are still possible such as thrombosis of the cannulated carotid and massive intracranial haemorrhages.

As for the last indication of moderate hypothermia which is the *treatment of cranio-cerebral injuries* and *of the most severe postoperative comas (therapeutic hypothermia)*, I would come to the following conclusions: from the data reported here by Prof. *Lazorthes*, it seems evident that, on the basis of a large clinical experience, he is convinced of the advantages of this method. Nevertheless from his own discussion, many debatable points are raised so that the problem cannot be considered definitely clear. I think that better than come to some definitive conclusions, we should make a sort of balance between positive and negative factors.

In favour of the use of therapeutic hypothermia are mainly the sound experimental data presented by *Rosomoff*.

It has to be however pointed out that *Rosomoff* states that the interval between lesion to the brain and beginning of cooling is necessarly limited to less than 8 hours.

In favour of therapeutic hypothermia are also many other Authors who, mainly from clinical impressions on groups more or less numerous of patients, are convinced of the advantages of the method.

I think that among the negative factors which limit or even exclude this indication of moderate hypothermia, the following are the most important:

a) timing: *Lazorthes* agrees on two substantial points: severely injured patients usually are taken to our Centers many hours or even days after the trauma and that hypothermia is difficult to maintain for more than three or four days. According therefore to *Rosomoff*'s experimental data, most of these patients theoretically should not have any advantage from the treatment which furthermore can be continued for a period of time definitely inferior to the duration of the most severe symptoms, which from our experience seldom clear before one week and sometimes may last much longer.

b) risk: *Lazorthes* emphasized that the use of the necessary drugs for induction and maintainance of hypothermia needs special caution and technical ability and that because of its complexity and the necessity of continuous controls, this method can *only* be used in some highly specialized centers.

c) the third negative factor is finally the lack of comparable series. Against the clinical impressions reported by *Lazorthes* and other Authors who are in favour, there are many others who think that hypothermia is unnecessary or even harmful.

In conclusion I would like to support here, in front of this qualified audience, the stimulating suggestion made by Prof. *Lazorthes:* let us initiate on a large scale and on strictly statistical basis, a coordinate study which will eventually enable us to establish the role of therapeutic hypothermia in the difficult but emotional field of neurosurgical resuscitation.

Druck: Steyrermühl, Wien VI.